A Guide to Digestive Disorders

(Complete Stomach and Bowel Care)

Published by :
Lotus Press Publishers & Distributors

A Guide to Digestive Disorders

(Complete Stomach and Bowel Care)

Dr. Rajeev Sharma
M.D., D.Lit.

Lotus PRESS

4735/22, Prakash Deep Building
Ansari Road, Darya Ganj,
New Delhi - 110002

Lotus Press : Publishers & Distributors
Unit No. 220, 2nd Floor, 4735/22, Prakash Deep Building,
Ansari Road, Darya Ganj, New Delhi- 110002
Ph.: 98118-38000
• E-mail : lotuspress1984@gmail.com
www.lotuspress.co.in

A Guide to Digestive Disorders

ISBN: 81-8382-161-8

Printed & Published by : **Lotus Press Publishers & Distributors,** New Delhi-02

About The Author

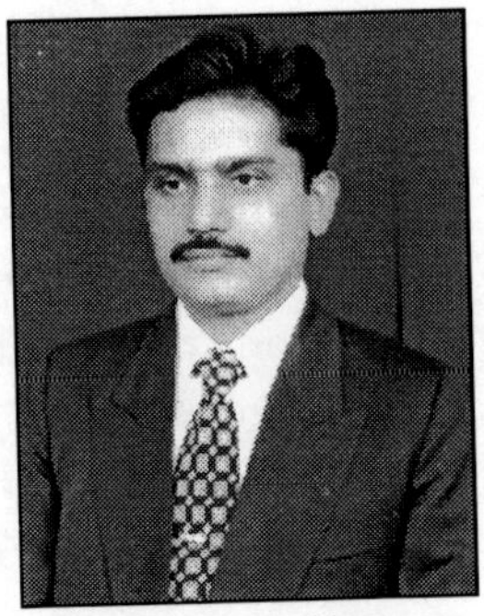

Dr. Rajeev Sharma

Dr. Rajeev Sharma is an eminent consultant of Homoeo-pathy, Yoga, Naturopathy and Alternative Medicine in India. He has written more than two hundred twenty five books (225) in Hindi and English and around one thousand articles which have been published in various newspapers and magazines. He is also an Editorial Board Member of the prestigious Asian Homoeopathic Journal besides many other newspapers and magazines.

Dr. Rajeev Sharma has written books on ayurveda, homoeo-pathy, yoga, naturopathy, accupressure, magnetotherapy, water-therapy, massage and aromatherapy etc., and on all major ailments.

Dr. Rajeev Sharma is Medical Advisor to Ralson Remedies (a homoeopathic manufacturer), and Dixit Pharmacy (Ayurvedic Manufacturer), Sr. Medical Officer U.P. Govt. He has received several prizes for his outstanding achievements. He has been awarded the *Best Author Prize in Hindi* by the Ministry of Health and Family Welfare, Government of India and *Sarjana Puraskar* by *U.P. Hindi Sansthan*, Lucknow. He has delivered talks on All India Radio and Total T.V. and lectures on Alternative Medicine in various Government and Non-government Organisations. He has written Advertisement for the products of several companies.

He has established an institute through which you can get certificates by correspondence in Accupressure, Massage, Yoga, Water Therapy, Diet Therapy, Naturopathy, Colour Therapy and Reiki besides other paramedical courses.

He is providing literature on Personality Development and Life-Style Management.

Dr. Rajeev Sharma is also a social activist. He has worked a lot against Addiction and Prevention of AIDS. He has worked for population and pollution control and human rights and has received the World Human Rights Promotion Award. His name has been published in *LIMCA BOOK OF RECORDS,* 2005. He has developed a website too:- www.newkamasutra.com

Dr. Rajeev Sharma is National President of an NGO UTKRISHTA BHARAT (An All India Association of Socio-Cultural—Religious and Sports Activities).

Preface

This book elaborates almost all the ailments of digestion including constipation, diarrohea, dysentry, hepatitis, hemorhoids, irritable bowel syndrome, acidity, nausea etc. The foods and nutrients required for body and helpful tables are also included in this book.

There are separate chapters on constipation, stomachache and abdominal pain. Treatment by naturopathy, yoga, ayurvedic medicines and homoeopathic medicines are also provided here for the benefit of readers.

To avoid digestive disorders one should take care of overeating, time of eating, items of eating and much more.

Food is meant of generate energy in the body so as to enable each and every body organ to discharge its individual functions. About eating we must not overlook or ignore undernoted points:

(i) Eat only when one is real hungry.

(ii) Eat daily at a fix time.

(iii) Diet should include cereals, pulses, seasonal green and leafy vegetables, fruits, fats (in moderate quantity), milk and milk products etc. In a way daily diet should be a balanced and nutritious diet, consisting of above mentioned food items which should also be rich in minerals and vitamins.

(iv) Avoid foods that cause constipation, loose motions, acidity, flatulence, abdominal colic, sour and acidic eructations, belching etc.

(v) Avoid foods which are fried and rich in condiments.

(vi) Use only unsturated Vegetable oils like, Soyabean, Sun-flower, Palm, Cotton seed oil etc. which reduce cholesterol level.

(vii) Avoid using clarified butter, oil, coconut oil, lard, olive oils and butter which raise cholesterol level, thus causing high blood pressure, cardiac disorders, obesity, joint pains and immobility.

(viii) Dietary fibre, obtained from whole grains, vegetables, and fruits should be used in sufficient quantity. Diet, rich in fibre content, is capable of reducing food intake, as it imparts a sense of satiation to the body.

Gluttons must resist the temptation of eating every time. It disturbs the digestive systems and denies rest to digestive organs and other body organs.

Hope readers will find it useful.

Dr. Rajeev Sharma

Srijan—Aarogya Jyoti®
Palm—11/03, Shipra Sun City
Ghaziabad (U.P.)
Ph.: 0120-6460127
email: sharmarajeev108@rediffmail.com

Contents

About The Author *v*

Preface *vii*

1. Essential Food Nutrients 1
2. Constipation and its Treatment 13
3. Abdominal Pain and its Treatment 19
4. Stomach Ache and Gas with Treatment Plan 21
5. Irritable Bowel Syndrome (I.B.S.) 23
6. Food for Digestive System 35
7. Common Digestive Disorders 36
   Constipation, Diarrhea, Dysentery, Nausea And Vomiting, Flatulent Colic/ Gas/Wind, Acidity and Heart Burn, Peptic Ulcer (Ulcer of Stomach), Jaundice, Cirrhosis of Liver, Hepatitis, Worms, Cancer of Stomach, Piles
8. Naturopathy—to Cure Digestive Disorders 52
9. Yoga—to Cure Different Digestive Disorders 67
10. Six Yogic Kriyas—to Cure Different Digestive Disorders 76
11. Juice Fast for Detoxification and Digestive Disorders 90
12. Ayurvedic Medicines for Different Digestive Disorders 96
13. Homeopathic Medicines for Different Digestive Disorders 114
14. Allopathic Treatment of Different Digestive Disorders 119
15. Physical Activities—to Cure Different Digestive Disorders 130
16. Calories, Height-Weight and Essential Nutrients Tables 141

1

ESSENTIAL FOOD NUTRIENTS

All foods are rich in various nutrients, as no single food item is an all-contained item that can give essential nutrients to a person to meet his daily requirements thereof. In order to have balanced diet, certain vegetables, fruits, cereals, dairy products, poultry products are required to be blended or not taken in isolation, except when a particular situation demands. Following nutrients are said to be essential ingredients of a balanced diet:

(*i*) Carbohydrates	(Sugar, wheat, grains, jaggery etc.)
(*ii*) Proteins	(Fish, grains, soyabeans, cheese, etc.)
(*iii*) Fats	(Saturated and unsaturated fats as butter, clarified butter, vegetable oils)
(*iv*) Vitamins	(A, B complex, C, D, E, K)
(*v*) Calcium	(Milk)
(*vi*) Minerals	(Iron, phosphorus, manganese, potassium, etc.)
(*vii*) Dietary Fibre	

Carbohydrates: These are components of oxygen, hydrogen and carbon. They provide energy and heat to our body. Sugar and starch are well known sources of energy and both of which exist in green plants. Starch causes accumulation of fat in the body and it is difficult to digest, thus straining the liver. Lack of carbohydrates causes weakness, run-down condition and restlessness in the body, whereas its excess causes fatness (obesity). Liver retains them in the form of glycogen which is released by it, as soon as body requires it to sustain energy. Excessive release of glycogen into blood stream can cause rise in sugar levels of the blood and depressed or deficient supply can often result in low sugar percentage in the blood, both being forms of diabetes known as hyper and hypoglycaemia respectively. A normal daily need of a person is 160 to 240 gms of carbohydrate which, often, is liable to vary depending on health status of a person.

Proteins: Proteins are required for proper development of our body and the word protein means 'first in importance'. They are conglomerates of phosphorus, sulphur, carbon, oxygen, nitrogen, etc. and deficient supply of proteins to the body will compel the body to eat its own muscles so that all vital organs do continue to function in a normal way. Main function of proteins is to grow, repair and maintain organs and tissues of the body. In order to facilitate assimilation of proteins, the body releases amino acids which are more than 70 in numbers. Enzymes break the proteins into amino acids which, in turn, help protein to get absorbed into the blood stream. Out of 70 amino acids, 10 are considered essential for the purpose and are known as high quality proteins. Chief sources of proteins are eggs, milk, soyabeans, almonds, nuts, fish and meats. Certain pulses, seeds, cereals, peas also contain protein but in a limited quantity. Pulses augment short supply of protein received from cereals. Hence, to get an added advantage, cereals, should always be taken with pulses.

Our skin, muscles, hormones and enzymes are composed of amino acids. Since their requirements are of permanent nature, so is the need for constant supply of proteins. In the absence or short supply of proteins to the body, one is liable to feel tired and weak, whereas their excess supply will vitiate our blood, as also let them rot in our intestines.

Daily requirement of protein of a person should be one gm per kg of body weight but it may be ensured that quality of protein is not inferior or substandard. For vegetarians, soyabeans are capable of giving almost double the amount of protein which an equal amount of fish can give. Is their any other bargain, in this respect, cheaper?

Fats: Fats discharge the function of lubricating the body, apart from being a concentrated source of energy and providing essential fatty acids for the aforesaid purpose. Our body's fat requirement is met from oils, pure fats. Apart from that some oil seeds, nuts, soyabean also supply fats. Pulses and cereals have meagre percentage of fats. It is a myth and a misplaced conception to totally eliminate oils from our diet. In fact, fats should form an essential part of our diet, as overuse is as dangerous and risky as total lack there of.

All oils and fatty acids have 3 types of fatty acids such as saturated (which are causatives of high rise of cholesterol in blood, if taken in excess), polysaturated acids do not raise cholesterol levels whereas monosaturated acids lower the level of cholesterol. Hydrogenated vanaspati oils are rich in saturated fatty acids and it also matters as to how and in what way they have been processed. Following table will clearly indicate the concentration of approximated quantity (percentage) in each variety of oil derived from various derivatives.

Oil	**%age of saturated fatty acids**	**% age of mono unsaturated fatty acids**	**% age of poly unsaturated fatty acids**
Butter oil	65	31	4
Coconut oil	91	6	3
Corn oil	13	26	61
Cotton Seed oil	28	19	53
Lard	43	45	12
Olive oil	14	77	9
Palm oil	53	37	10
Peanut oil	18	49	33
Sesame oil	16	41	43
Soyabean oil	16	24	60
Sunflower oil	11	22	67
Safflower oil	11	12	77

For a normal adult daily consumption of fat, from 25-35 gms, seems to be in order. Persons, doing hard and strenuous work, would require higher quantity of fat which should mainly be had from polyunsaturated fats, preferably vegetables. Heat generated by fats is almost double the amount of energy generated by carbohydrates, when process of oxidation takes place in the body. This energy is converted into body-heat and muscular work. Patients, who suffer from heart ailments, arteriosclerosis, high blood pressure or any other similar disorder, should avoid saturated fats and substitute them with poly unsaturated fats. They should also avoid lard, palm oil, cream, butter. Instead they should lay stress on the use of skimmed milk and its bi-products.

Vitamins: Vitamins are essential ingredients of food. They assist carbohydrates, fats, proteins and other nutrients to promote various chemical processes, increase energy, replace and build cells . For maintaining good health, vitamins serve as protective foods. Following vitamins have, so far, been isolated.

Vitamin A: Its deficiency results in lack of appetite, night blindness, retarded growth, unhealthy skin, dental loss, depleted vitality and general growth. Its natural sources are fruits, vegetables, egg yolk, milk and its products, liver oil and liver of animals. In normal health one requires 5000 I.V. daily but in pregnancy and for lactating (nursing) mothers 8000 I.U. will do because its deficiency can lead to deficiency in milk secretion.

Vitamin B-I (Thiamine): Thiamine deficiency leads to depressed mental states, nervous irritation, weight loss, tickling sensation in the soles. It is of paramount importance for functions of muscles, nervous system, digestion, for promoting utilization of carbohydrates. Its daily normal requirement is 1.25 mg. It is derived from natural sources like peanuts, oatmeal, milk, rice husk, brewer's yeast, meat, liver etc.

Vitamin B-2 (Riboflavin): It promotes growth and general health, is useful for fine conditions of skin and eyes, helps body cells in using oxygen for release of energy from food and its deficiency may result in cracking of lip-corners and burning/ itching of eyes. Its natural sources are milk and its products, whole grains, meat, liver and various foods. Its daily requirement, for a normal person, is 150 mg.

Vitamin B-6 (Pyridoxine): Its presence is essential in adding assimilation of proteins and fats, in blood building for normal functioning of brain, muscles and nervous system but its deficiency often results in disorders of nervous system, loss of hair, skin eruptions, loss of muscular control etc., Milk, banana, raisins, molasses, wheat germ, brain, brewers yeast, kidney, liver, fish, eggs, meats are natural sources of vitamin B-6. Its daily requirement is 2.0 mg.

Vitamin B-12 (Cobalamin) : It helps is promoting growth of children, helps as a general tonic for the aged persons, in regenerating and forming R.B.Cs (Red Blood Corpuscles), nerve tissue and also in utilization of carbohydrates, fats and proteins. Its deficiency often leads to lack of proper growth, inflammation of tongue (though quite occasional), fatigue and anaemia. Its natural sources are eggs, liver, meats, milk products, etc. Its daily requirement is 6.0 mg daily, in normal course.

Vitamin B-5 (Pantothenic acid): Deficiency of this vitamin is often not found but, when it occurs, it may cause dizzy spells and disturbance in digestion. It is considered necessary for synthesis of antibiotics, nervous and digestive system. Its natural sources are brain, whole wheat, brewer's yeast, molasses, peas, kidney, liver etc. Said to blacken hair (not medically proved). For daily requirement 10 mg would suffice.

Vitamin-C (Ascorbic Acid): It builds up general resistance of the body, enabling the latter to fight infection, apart from hastening heeling. It is essential for healthy bones, teeth and gums, maintains vigour and good health, in restricting coughs, colds and sneezing. Its deficiency can lead to anaemia, bleeding from piles, lack of general resistance, etc. All citrus fruits are its major sources as also amla, mango, lime, lemon, tomatoes, potatoes, peppers, spinach and other vegetables and fruits. If stored or cooked, it is liable to be destroyed. Its daily normal requirement is 60 mg but may be required more in case of smoking, incessant sneezing and coryza. It may have to be increased to 500 mg daily, depending on severity and gravity of the case.

Vitamin-D (Calciferol) : It helps in the formation of bones and teeth for utilization of phosphorus and calcium. Its deficiency leads to rickets in infants and children. In pregnancy puffiness and swelling of feet, etc. indicate its deficiency, caused by malabsorption of calcium. Ultraviolet rays help to convert cholesterol, present in the skin, to calciferol. Its natural sources are milk, milk products, oil of fish and liver. Excess of this vitamin may cause toxic effects. Its daily requirement, for a normal person, is 400 I.U. But far higher dosage is required in pregnancy. Should never be used without medical advice and care.

Vitamin -E (Tocopherol): It helps in prevention of undesirable blood clots, and promotes formation of new skin (in the women). Its deficiency can lead to early ageing, muscular disorders, loss of reproductive capacity. Its natural sources are wheat germ, grain and its products, leaf and green vegetables, margarine, vegetable oils, liver, eggs and butter and its daily requirement is 30 I.U. if situation demands. As for its importance, only vitamin C can be given with it.

Vitamin-K (Menadione): It assists in maintaining clotting system of blood. But for this vitamin and its capability to prevent clotting in blood, even a simple injury could have lead to fatality. For healthy and efficient working of liver it has an important part to play. It is found in wheat, brain, wheat germ, tomatoes, cabbages, potatoes, spinach, liver and egg-yolk. Bacteria, present in the human intestines, produces this vitamin, hence it hardly needs to be supplemented, but its use and importance cannot be overlooked or denied.

Note: We have mentioned only very prominent and generally used vitamins. In addition, there are other vitamins like Niacin, Folic acid, Biotin, Vitamin F, Vitamin P (Bioflavonoid), Vitamin B-15.

Best course is to extract vitamins from vegetables and fruits and tablets or tonics should be taken only when the body is unable to extract vitamins from natural foods. All vitamins, falling under B-Complex category, are water-soluble and, thus, are drained out by system. If too much of vitamins are taken continuously for longer periods, it may render our body incapable of drawing vitamins from natural foods.

Minerals

There are five basic (or gross) minerals for the body such as, calcium, phosphorus, potassium, sodium and magnesium and trace elements consist of iron, copper, iodine, chromium, zinc and manganese, besides selenium. In addition, cobalt, nickle, sulphur, fluorine and gases (like oxygen, carbon, hydrogen and nitrogen). All such elements play an important part in physical well-being of the body, enabling it to discharge its functions efficiently. Calcium is meant for bones, iron for blood- building, iodine for warding off goitre and manganese to reduce risk of cancer, improper balance between chromium and manganese may lead to heart disorders. If zinc is deficient, it is likely to lead to sexual dysfunction, anorexia (loss of appetite) and alopecia (baldness or loss of hair from the head).

Due to lack or deficient supply of minerals to our system certain physical upsets can be discerned. A brief account of important minerals is given below.

Calcium: It helps to form and maintain teeth and bones, blood to clot, in regulating cardiac rhythm and helps normal contraction of muscles. Calcium provides endurance and vitality, modifies menstrual pains, fortifies nerves. It also dispels depressed moods, loss of sleep, allergies of various origins, irritability of temper. Calcium deficiency is common in aged persons, menopausal state, smokers, etc. For absorption of calcium, vitamin C and D are required. Its natural sources are milk and its products, leafy and green vegetables, citrus fruits, peanuts, beans, sunflower seeds, soybeans, pulses, etc. If calcium deficiency is not made up from the above and other sources, the body takes up calcium from a person's bones. Calcium in conjunction with magnesium, helps in maintaining well-being of cardiovascular system.

Phosphorus: It is required for normal structure of teeth and bones and also for changing food enzymes into energy. It helps in absorption of calcium but, if in excess, it can make calcium uptake difficult. Phosphorus deficiency manifests itself in the form of general debility, pain in bones and lowered appetite. It helps to excrete, promote nervous health, hasten the healing process, and does not let calcium escape from the site of injury. Fat rich diet and crystal sugar help to maintain proper phosphorus. Calcium balance, whereas excess of magnesium/ iron can block storage of phosphorus. Important sources of phosphorus are milk and milk products, seeds, nuts, fish, egg, poultry, meet, bread and whole grain cereals, pulses, beans, etc. Its supply to bone is adversely affected if antacids are used. It should never be taken by anyone of one's own, except under medical supervision.

Potassium: Life would not have been possible without potassium which is a key mineral. Whole body chemistry is liable to be disturbed if body were to take it from the cells. Its deficiency will create a craving in pregnant women to eat clay/chalk. Its deficiency can cause weakness in muscle, irregular heart-beats, and irritable temperament but, its excess can cause various heart irregularities. It is essential for maintaining normal functions of nerves, muscles, cardiac functions and enzyme reactions, apart from regulating and balancing body fluids. Advancing age demands potassium in greater quantity for getting over muscle fatigue, inability to relax, constipation, itching on skin, nausea and cramps in the muscles. If such symptoms surface even in younger persons, it indicates deficiency of potassium. Higher intake of potassium can lead walls of blood vessels free from calcium deposits. Apple cider vinegar is an excellent source of potassium which (one tsp mix with a glass of water), if sipped slowly, will emulsify fat, reduce high blood pressure, may also improve joints mobility. It (potassium) does not let sodium raise the blood pressure. Potassium deficiency could easily be prevented by a cup of coffee or alcohol in moderate quantity. It will also modify symptoms arising out of diarrhoea, liver torpidity, sweating or excessive use of diuretics. Its usual sources are dates, wheat germ, potatoes, cabbage, peas, peanuts, dried powder of skimmed milk, seeds, fish and poultry but, above all, from apple cider vinegar. Its daily intake is about 275 gms daily. More intake of sodium will increase loss of potassium, from inside the body cells.

Manganese: It helps in proper utilization of vitamins B and E by activating various enzymes. It helps to remove indigestion and fatigue, helps blood clotting process and also produces more milk in nursing mothers. Since it increases glucose tolerance, it is useful in diabetes also. Its excessive intake will badly affect absorption of iron. Though its deficiency is hardly found in human beings, it can be easily obtained from whole grain bran, seeds, nuts, shell-fish, organ meats and black tea.

Magnesium: It is found in each cell of human body. Imbalance between calcium and magnesium ratio can affect nervous system. Though our body contains hardly 50gms of it but, even then, its importance cannot be denied or overlooked. It helps to metabolize vitamin E and calcium. Its low content may even cause cancer, apart from causing diabetes. Vitamin B-6 and magnesium are known to have reduced risks of gall-bladder and kidney stones. It is found in abundance in hard water and those who drink hard water are reported to have negligible number of heart attacks. Strenuous physical exercises account for its depletion, often resulting in weakness, muscular contraction. It can be obtained from pulses, grain cereals, green and leafy vegetables, sea-food, dairy products and cereals, apart from hard water, as mentioned above.

Sodium: It assists in maintaining water-balance, inside and outside cells of the body. If taken in excess, it can trigger up blood pressure, cancer of liver, congestive cardiac disorders, renal diseases, but its deficiency can result in oedema, cramps in muscles. It is lost from our body through sweat and urine.

It is not easily obtained from the content of sodium found in foods, hence its deficiency is made up by common table salt (Sodium chloride). Its excessive intake is far more dangerous than its depletion which can be easily compensated from meats, processed food and sodium itself.

Zinc: Zinc performs lots of functions, either alone or in conjunction with other factors. It handles functioning of protein and carbohydrates and aids in normal functioning of tissues. Too much use of alcohol, food refining, low-protein diet, pregnancy, cold and diseases can cause its deficiency which, in turn, can lead to retarded growth process, loss of appetite and taste, delayed healing of wounds, lack of sexual maturity and dysfunction of reproductive system. Intestines are equipped to dispose of extra quantity of zinc which the body does not require. As the age advances, zinc deficiency may occur. Zinc is found in plenty from processed cheese, brewer's east, nuts, seeds, brain, wheat germ, rice (brown in particular), spinach, cottage cheese, poultry eggs and sea food, whole grains. Flour of whole wheat and its products contain four times more zinc, as compared to white flour.

Apart from the aforesaid minerals there are others too, like lead, aluminium, cadmium and mercury which are heavy metals but are not so significant as the above mentioned ones.

Dietary Fibre: It is the component that makes the cell walls in the plants and is non-digestible, due to the fact that it cannot be broken down by body enzymes nor can it be absorbed by the body and, perhaps due to this very reason, it was thought to have no dietary value and, thus, discarded. But the said conception was wrong as it implied that it had no mechanical properties, But it has the capacity to trap water and to keep the faeces moistened, thus removing constipation. But for the dietary fibre intestines would never have been able to expel faecal matter, thus reducing the risk of accumulation of toxic substances and inflammation in the intestines.

Barley, oats, legumes and fruits have rich soluble fibre content, whereas wheat and most other cereals and vegetables have more insoluble fibre in them. The former help to lower serum cholesterol level but raise good cholesterol HDL, but the latter relieve constipation and improve digestion.

To affect reduction in weight, high fibre diets are more useful, for it takes much longer to chew them, gives more satisfaction to the eater, requires expense of more energy, reduces appetite and are stomach-friendly as they provide sense of fullness. Fibre helps in formation of stool, renders it bulkier and softer. The more the bulk and softness, the easier it is for the intestines to expel them. That is why cabbage and carrots are a preferred choice for those who wish to remain free from costive bowels. Bed-ridden patients should not take high fibre diets. A high fat-diet is always a low-fibre diet and high fibre diet is always a low-fat diet as "A high fibre diet tends to lower the blood pressure of hypersensitive persons."

Cholesterol: It is a yellow-white, waxy element produced mostly in the liver, and is a master molecule that plays an important role in lives of all beings. It is like a building block that the body uses to make other elements in the body. It is essential for the survival of human life. Cholesterol is part and parcel of muscles, fat tissues, brain and nerves and, if it is between 140-160 mg, it is said to be within normal limits in a normal healthy person. It is generated by diet and is active in metabolic processes of blood plasma, liver and intestines. Serum cholesterol level beyond 240 mg is high, below 240 mg and up to 20 mg tolerable, and from 160-200 mg is ideal.

It is triggered and precipitated by risk factors, like high blood pressure, smoking, obesity, diabetes, disorder of circulation, sedentary life and lack of physical activity, heredity, more in male gender and aged persons- all these factors are held to cause fall in low HDL (High density lipoproteins). It is the LDL that is the chief factor (low density Lipoproteins) for causing calcareous and crustaceous deposits in the arteries which, in turn, block the passage of blood. Efforts should always be made to raise HDL through diet and thus, lower LDL level. LDL can be effectively lowered by soluble fibre obtained from sunflower seeds, pectin (found in apples and citrus fruits) and corn, in addition to niacin, chromium, magnesium, oat bran, dry beans, etc. (which are other sources to lower LDL and raise HDL).

Of all the contributory causes, saturated fats are the major sources for raising cholesterol levels in the blood. So, consumption of red meats, chicken, whole milk, dry fruit should be avoided. Lack of exercise, sedentary habits, gluttony, obesity are other causes. Let fruits and vegetables play an important role in dietary menus of each home.

■

2

CONSTIPATION AND ITS TREATMENT

Constipation is a condition in which the bowels are evacuated at a longer interval or with difficulty. What the right interval should be, is difficult to generalize since it varies from person to person. Some evacuate their bowels once, others twice a day, while there are others who seek this pleasure only once in 2 or 3 days and yet have sound health.

What Causes Constipation?

Some may have constipation on account of the change of enviornment, or emotional tension, but the normal rhythm returns after a few days, and should not be a source of worry. The most important causes of constipation are a disregard of the call to pass motion and an improper diet. When the rectum is full, it sends signals to the intestines through the central nervous system for their movement and if this is repeatedly ignored it gradually leads to failure of the rectum to signal the urge. The diet should contain a reasonable amount of non absorbable material to form a bulk which acts as a stimulus for the intestinal movements. Highly spicy food such as *chaat*, pickles and hot curries may stimulate the bowel to cause a complete evacuation, but this is followed by inactivity of the intestines and constipation. Slimilarly, purgatives also stimulate the intestines, to cause their evacuation and this is also followed by constipation. To treat this constipation, again a purgative is needed and this continues in the form of a constipation purgative constipation cycle. Other causes of constipation may be a disease or abnormality of gastrointestinal tract, adverse effects of drugs, drying of the stools (faecal impaction), obstruction of the intestines, and severe illness in which food intake is too small.

In case of prolonged constipation in the infants or intermittent constipation with diarrhoea, the physician should be consulted to rule out surgical problems.

What Can Be Done About Constipation?

If you are suffering from constipation, and have been taking purgative, try to stop these gradually. Your system will probably return to normal if you take enough soups, vegetables, fruits etc. However, if you are the worrying type you may take milk laxative only as a temporary measure without making it a habit. Remember, disregarding the call for motion is the worst you can do to your consipation. Do not wait unnecessarily. Rush to the toilet wherever you are, whether at a party or in the kitchen. Your diets should be made up of high roughage foods containing a lot of whole grain cereals, leafy vegetables like spinach, raw carrots and cucumbers, salads, prunes, figs, papaya, water melon and other fresh fruits. Your intestines will soon gain the normal tone. If all these measures fail, you are a candidate for milk purgatives or laxatives. Never take strong purgatives. They are needed only under exceptional circumstances and should be used under the care of a doctor. The purgatives which are commonly used are described here.

Mild Purgatives

Mild purgatives or laxatives are those which promote defecation causing minimum adverse effects. Drugs included in this group are:

Bulk Producing Drugs

Isapgol (sat Isabgol), Agar-agar (Agarol), Methyle celluslose.

These drugs absorb water to increase the bulk in the intestines and make the stools soft. The onset of their action is slow, about 12 to 24 hours. They are the safest purgatives for the treatment of chronic constipation. Of the three, isapgol is most commonly used in our country.

Dosage

Isapgol is given preferably with warm milk in a dose of 4 to 5 g once or twice a day. Agar-agar is given in a dose of 4 to 16 g and methyl cellulose in 1 to 6 g in divided doses, for children in the age group of 12-15 years. For younger children the dose should be half.

Adverse Effects

Those agents which are derived from vegetable sources are devoid of toxic effects. Occasionally flatulence may occur, but, this can be relieved by increasing the fluid intake. The chronic use of isapgol may decrease plasma cholesterol by interfering with the absorption of bile acids but it does not cause any harm and may rather do good to an obese patient.

Precaution

Always take plenty of fluids along with these drugs to obtain maximum benefit and to avoid the possibility of intestinal obstruction which has been reported to occur in rare cases.

Stool Softeners

Dioctyle Sodium Sulfosuccinate

This is an effective stool softener for the treatment of constipation in some cases. It is a detergent which absorbs water by reducing the surface tension of fluids in the stools.

Dosage

The daily dose varies from 50 to 500mg depending on the severity of the condition. The action starts after 24 to 48 hours.

Adverse Effects

Adverse effects of this drug are quite rare. It has been reported to interact with mineral oils to increase their absorption.

Precaution

It should not be taken with mineral oils.

Liquid Paraffin (Cremaffin)

This is a traditional remedy for constipation. It is an inert oil which lubricates the intestines and forms a film or coating around the stools to make its passage smooth and comfortable. It softens the stool by preventing the absorption of water into the intestines. It is often recommended to patients of piles, heart attack, and to pregnant women, as well as after surgery on the rectum or abdomen and in cases in which straining to evacuate may be harmful. It is quite popular as it allows the stool to pass through the intestines with a minimum of friction.

Dosage

Liquid paraffin is given in a dose of 15 to 45 ml. Its action starts after 12 to 24 hours.

Adverse Effects

If taken regularly, it may cause deficiency of fat soluble Vitamins such as A, D and K. It may at times leak through the gastrointestinal tract and cause not only annoying but embarrassing situation. Its presence in the rectum inhibits the stimulatory reflexes to the intestines and prevents complete evacuation of bowels. On aspiration, liquid paraffin has also been reported to cause lipoid pneumonia in elderly and weak persons. Although it promotes and facilitates the passage of stools, it delays healing and, therefore, its use is not preferred after surgery for piles.

Precautions

1. It should not be taken regularly as it may cause deficiency of Vitamins A, D and K. This may be very harmful, specially in pregnant women.
2. It should not be taken by very old and weak persons, and young children because of the danger of lipoid pneumonia.

3. It should not be taken during the day time because of chances of its leakage through the rectum.
4. It delays healing, and is not recommended after an operation on piles.
5. It should not be taken along with dioctyls sodium sulfosuccinate, as the latter promotes its absorption from the intestines.

Mild Saline Purgatives

Magnesium Hydroxide

This is a mild laxative which can be used even by pregnant women and children. It absorbs water from the intestines to form the bulk and make the stools soft. Besides purgative action, it counteracts acidity in the stomach.

Dosage

Its usual dose is 2 to 4g. its action starts after 2 to 6 hours.

Adverse Effects

It is a mild purgative and does not have any adverse effect except to produce flatulence in some people.

Precautions

1. Take plenty of fluids along with this purgative.
2. Patients with chronic kidney disease who may have difficulty excreting magnesium should be wary of milk of Magnesia.

Sodium Potassium Tartrate

It is the basic ingredient of commonly used ENO's fruit salt and Seidlitz powder. These also contain tartaric acid and sodium bicarbonate which interact to produce carbondioxide gas, forming an effervescen drink, which resembles gas containing soft drinks. The gas present in the solution distends the stomach and reflexly stimulates movements of the intestines. It also absorbs water from the intestines which assists in forming the bulk and softening the stools.

Dosage

The dose of sodium potassium tartrate for its purgative action is 10g. Its action starts after 3 to 6 hours.

Adverse Effects

Sodium potassium tartrate is a safe purgative and does not cause any adverse effect.

Precautions

It should not be taken by those who are on a sodium restricted diet, e.g. patients of heart failure, hypertension etc, but children are free of all such problems.

Important Note: The dose for children below the age of 8 years should be half of the prescribed dose and always consult with your paediatrician before taking this medicine.

■

3

ABDOMINAL PAIN AND ITS TREATMENT

Abdominal pain, one of the most frequently occurring symptoms, may originate from any organ in the abdomen, like the stomach, intestines, appendix, gall bladder, pancreas and kidneys. There are number of causes for this and therefore, any patient of abdominal pain of recent onset requires early and thorough evaluation for accurate diagnosis. However, the commonest source of abdominal pain in the region of stomach and intestines is the gastointestinal tract which consists of the stomach and intestines because it deals with outside material, i.e. the food and drink we take. A little overeating may cause distension and indigestion. A spicy meal may lead to an increase in acid secretion and sour eructations. In these conditions some digestives or antacids are taken for relief. Often flatulence, diarrhoea, dysentery, or an infection may produce spasms of the walls of the intestines causing a gripping type of pain called colic. This is a distressing situation and suitable measures for immediate relief are necessary.

Various household remedies like massage, hot water fomentation, *churan*, *ajwain*, *jaljeera*, and sometimes even purgatives are tried, but their success is usually limited. Therefore, the patient takes one of the preparations mentioned as pain killer which provides immediate relief. What is so special about these preparations that they provide such dramatic relief? It you look at the salts of any tablet, you will find that all the preparations contain an antispasmodic (which prevents spasm of the smooth muscle of the intestine). In addition, all these agents contain either a pain reliever or a sedative and some even contain a purgative. Such remedial measures may be effective in mitigating the colicky or intermittent type of pain. However, if it is frequent or of a dull constant nature, the physician must be consulted. Under such circumstances the continued and prolonged use of these drugs instead of improving the condition, may produce serious adverse effects. Since an antispasmodic is the most common ingredient of all these preparations, we will elaborate a little on it.

Antispasmodics

These are atropine or its synthetic substitute (anticholinergic drugs) and are used for relieving the spasm of the muscles of the intestine. The actions of almost all these drugs are more or less the same. There are only slight differences in their potency or duration of action. There may be some adverse effects caused and precautions to be observed with these drugs.

Combinations

After antispasmodics, the next common ingredient in all these preparations is a pain reliever. Some contain a sedative or a tranquillizer as well. Pain relievers may not be of much help unless the spasm is reduced. Undiagnosed pain precludes the use of phenolphthalein, a purgative, even if it is associated with constipation. Phenolphthalein itself aggravates gripping pain being irritant in nature. All these combinations have no greater value than the use of antispasmodics alone apart from increasing the cost and side effects. Some important drugs are Meftolspas, Proxyvon, Colimex, Cyclopam, Buscopan etc. In case of children use only after taking advice from your paediatrician.

■

4

STOMACH ACHE AND GAS WITH TREATMENT PLAN

The distress or stomach ache after eating is actually classified in two ways:

1. Distress appearing immediately after eating (postprandial distress): symptoms arise half an hour after a meal, such as abdominal bloating, distension, fullness or pressure.

2. Intestinal distress: Here symptoms usually start half an hour after eating and continue for several hours depending upon person to person. They may involve the stomach, small or large intestines with additional symptoms (to that of postprandial distress) such as abdominal pain and cramps and/or anal flatus.

Excess of gas in stomach and intestines is quite distressing and it is due to the disordered intestinal movements which delays the passages of gases through the bowel. Drugs might provide a symptomatic relief in the following ways:

1. The active ingredients may lower the surface tension of the stomach contents to facilitate the action of digestive juices, which will speed up the digestion and the passage of food contents from the stomach into the intestines.

2. The active ingredients may speed up stomach emptying by changing the stomach's acidity or increasing the contractions of smooth muscles of the stomach or by some other mechanisms.

The commonly available preparations, usually in combination, may contain the following ingredients:

Antiflatulents: Dimethicone (dimethypolysiloxane) and simethicone (a combination of dimethylpolysiloxanes and silica gel) act as antifoaming agent by reducing surface tension. The small mucous covered bubbles of gas (which hold air back) come close to each other, coalesce, and a large bubble is formed which is easily expelled out.

Carminative Oils: Peppermint, cumin, 'azovan' oils, etc. relax the muscles between oesophagus and stomach, increase the gastric secretions and churning in the stomach accelerate the passage of food from stomach.

Antacids: Magnesium trisilicate, light magnesium oxide, sodium carbonate etc. reduce gastric acidity.

Sodium Bicarbonate: It is a household baking soda (*mitha*-soda) which releases carbon dioxide as it interacts with acid in the stomach. It is useful for relieving distress after meal. Elderly patients above 60 should not consume more than a teaspoonful daily and if one is already on sodium or salt restricted diet, physician approval is necessary. In any case, this should not be used for more than a fortnight, unless a physican directs so.

Charcoal: Activated charcoal and wood charcoal can relieve bloating and other intestinal distress symptoms on account of its absorbent properties. However, it may bind a number of drugs and inactivate them for the same (absorbent) reason. Not more than 10g per day in divided doses would be safe for adults. So, for children the dose should be half.

■

5

IRRITABLE BOWEL SYNDROME (I.B.S.)

I.B.S is a functional disorder. It responds poorly to a biomedical philosophy of managment and must be understood in the context of the patient's psychological and social environment.

Aetiology of IBS

Irritable bowel disease is likely to be sub-divided into various groupings with different aetiologies.

Abnormal Gut Motility

Diarrhoea, constipation or a pattern altering between these two is characteristic of IBS, and led to the theory that intenstial dysmotility is the primary disorder. Pain and abdominal bloating which often accompany these symptoms, could then be due to enteric smooth muscle spasm and impaired intenstial clearance of gas.

This theory sounds plausible, but no distinctive pathophysiology of intestinal motor function has been identified. However, intenstial motility is complex and difficult to examine directly. It is possible that abnormal neuromuscular signalling, which cannot be detected by current technology, may be found in some patients with IBS.

Gut Hypersensitivity

There is more evidence supporting the theory that patients, with IBS have altered responsiveness to a range of afferent stimuli: they have supersensitive intestine. This effect is demonstrated by a crude but useful test for IBS which rectal distension with air during sigmoidoscopy can reproduce the patient's pain. This has been studied further using controlled hydrostatic distension of the colon by intraluminal ballons. Patients with IBS had a lower pain threshold than the control group.

A number of other stimuli have been found to produce gut symptoms at lowr thresholds in patients with IBS, including:

- Some mental and physical stressors;
- Gut peptides;
- Cholinergic stimuli;
- Bile acids;
- Dietary fats.

The evidence for afferent hypersensitivity is generally more compelling than for a primary motor disorder.

Psychosomatic cause

Most of them have some form of phychopathology. The most common diagnosis are anxiety and/or depression, yet the evidence that these are primary problems and that the gut sympotms are secondry is not very compelling-depression is slightly more likely than anxiety to be a primary problem.

A number of studies have measured psychological stress, and their results have supported many patients' self-reported experience that sympotms are worse at time of stress. However, more rigorous studies have found that the association is weaker than clinical experience suggests. Study results are inconsistent, and a recent multivariate analysis has actually found lower levels of stress in IBS patients than in controls! However, stressful life events probably increase the likelyhood of hospital referral.

Food Intolerance

Some patients with lactose intolerance secondry to mucosal hypolactasia have IBS-like symptoms, and may benefit from milk withdrawal. However, lactose deficiency is not increased in IBS.

Possible factors in irritable bowel disease.

- Primary disorder of gastrointenstinal motility
- Hypersensitivity of gut mucosa
- Psychological problem
- Food intolerance
- Specfic trigger
- Gastrointestinal infection
- Drugs
- Pelvic surgery

It has been suggested that there is a much larger group of patients with a wider range of food intolerance. Although there is no reliable laboratory or immunological test for food intolerance, doubleblind food challenges have identified patients with IBS whose symptoms improve if the offending foodstuff are excluded. However, this finding can only be regarded as indirect evidence for the role of food intolerance in the pathogenesis of IBS.

Specific Triggers

Some patients can link the onset of symptoms to external factors, such as gastroenteritis or antobiotics. Hysterectomy occasionally precipitates IBS in women.

There are certain life events too which may trigger IBS are:

- Death of a parent
- Leaving home
- Marriage

- Having children
- Break down of a relationship
- Unemployment
- An abusive experience

Clinical picture of IBS

The characterstic features of IBS are well known. The Manning criteria was the first attempt to diagnose IBS from the patient's history. They were derived from a study of a group of patients with IBS who were given a list of 15 sympotoms and asked which ones they had. Six symptoms were closely correlated with the diagnosis of IBS. The more symptoms a patient has, the more likely he is to have IBS.

Rome criteria for the diagnosis of IBS

At least three months' continuous or recurrent symptoms of Abdominal pain or discomfort which is

- Relieved with defaecation
- And/or associated with a change in frequency of stool
- and/or associated with a change in consistency of stool

And two or more of the following on at least a quarter of occasions or days;

- Altered stool frequency
- Altered stool
- Altered stool passage
- Bloating or feeling of abdominal distension

Other symptoms associated with IBS

- Indigetion
- Heart burn
- Tiredness

- Backache
- Headache
- Dizziness
- Breathlessness
- Frequent Urination

Minimum investigation for IBS

- Full blood count
- Erythrocyte sedimentation rate
- Multi-channel biochemistry
- Sigmoidoscopy
- Rectal biopsy (especially if patient has diarrhoea)

The reliability of Manning's criteria has been confirmed in subsequent studies. They have formed the basis for the Rome symptom criteria which are now used as diagnostic criteria for clinical studies.

Making the diagnosis

Patients presenting with bowel symptoms should have a thorough history and examination, as well as selective investigation. When taking the histrory, general practitioners should be aware of any factors that could increase the likelihood of the patient having a functional problem.

A prolonged series of tests can cause unnecessary anxiety. It is useful to tell the patient that the result of investigation are likely to be normal, so that the subsequent explanation that tests are normal becomes a positive experience. The minimum investigations usally performed are listed below:

INVSTIGATION GUIDELINES

It is difficult to formulate guidelines on when to proceed to barium enema or colonoscopy. With increasing experience and confidence, the need for the physician (as opposed to the patient) to be reassured declines.

The length of history and the age of the patient are the most common factors influencing the decision to image the colon. We tend to do a colonoscopy in patients with predominant diarrhoea, as this group has a greater chance of organic pathology than other patterns of altered bowel habit.

Dietary Advice

The traditional advice to eat a high-fibre diet may be good theoretically, but has proved to be virtually useless in many people. This lack of benefit has been confirmed by clinical studies.

Patients often ask for dietary advice and may offer a list of aggravating foodstuffs. There is no reason why they cannot try subtracting specific foods. Particularly committed patients may work through an exclusive. One can take the help of a dietician.

Summary

- Ten to fifteen percent of the population have symptoms of the irritable bowel syndrome, and the prevalence is higher in women.
- Although IBS has traditionally been a diagnosis of exclusion, modern management emphasizes the need to make a positive diagnosis.
- Patients with IBS who are referred to outpatient departments are more likely to be anxious and have neurotic symptoms than those treated in the community.
- It is probable that, as its genesis is better understood, IBS will be sub-divided into various groupings with differing aetiologies.
- Characterstic clinical features of IBS include abdominal pain, disturbance of bowel habit, bloating and passage of mucus per rectum.

- It is helpful to tell the patient that the result of investigations are likely to be normal, so that the subsequent explanation that tests are normal becomes a positive experience.
- Management should include a sympathetic explanation, a trial of diet, and constitutional symptomatic treatment.

Psychological Approaches

In addition to a conventional approach, counsellor, phychologist or psychiastrist may be consulted. Some patients seem to respond to hypnotheraphy.

Pschological Treatments Useful in IBS

- Hypnotherapy
- Cognitive Behavioural therapy
- Psychodynamic psychotherapy
- Anti depressents.

Excersises and Yoga

After every meal lie down first on your right side. Take deep breath eight times. Turn and lie down on your back and take 16 deep breaths, now turn on your left side and deep breathe 32 times.

Vajrasana, Padmasana, Parvatasana, Pavanamuktasana, Bhujangasasa, Dhanurasana, Matyasana and yogamudra are good for digestive disorder.

Hydrotherapy

Take a thin cloth, may be a hand-towel, of the required size according to the area of application. Dip it in ice cold water and squeeze out the water to prevent dripping. Frequent changing of the compres is necessary before it gets warm. In order to make the compress last longer, a thicker compress will serve better. It must be pressed frimely in place.

Very cold applications are given with ice chips filled in a rubber bag with screw cap. If ice-bag is not available, woollen or flannel can be used instead. The pack must not drip. The area to be treated must be covered with a towel and the pack should be placed above it. This is useful for abdominal pain.

Hip Bath

Hip bath is given mainly for abdominal disorders. It can be given sitting in an ordinary bath tub with the legs on the sides of the tub or in a tub which can accommodate a person to sit comfortably with the legs resting on the floor.

Procedure

Fill the tub with hot water enough to cover the hip. The temperature of the water should be as per the individual's tolerance. A brisk massage should be given frequently to the abdomen as long as one is in the bath. The duration of the bath can be from 5-15 minutes. After coming out of the bath splash or spray cold water and dry-briskly with a coarse towel. Hot hip bath is useful in constipation, piles, obesity, distended stomach, poor digestion and worms.

A cold hip bath can be given similarly for better circulation of the internal organs of the abdomen, and for the same duration. At the end of the bath do not splash or spray water but give a vigorous rub with a thick towel and scrub dry.

Cold hip bath is useful for the same disorders as hot hip bath when used alternating the former.

Internal bath

Enema is the water treatment given to the bowels and rectum. Giving enema in all diseases is an essential part of naturopathy.

The uncleared morbid substance inside the bowels is effectively removed by enema. When the bowels are clean, the severtity of the disease automatically reduces. By taking enema the muscle tone of the bowels and rectum increases and its healthy movement is restored.

For perfect cleansing, enema is preferably given in the morning after the evacuation. However, in cases of constipation, enema is given first thing in the morning.

Enema is given in three convential positions, lying down on the left side, lying on the back with knees raised and stooping forward in a standing position with knees bent. A thorough cleansing cannot be obtained in the squatting position or sitting on toilet bowl.

Method of giving enema

Assume the desired position. Suspend the enema pot filled with half a litre of pure tap water, one metre above. Apply a little oil or vaseline to the nozzle of the rectal tube. Before insertion check the rectal tube to ensure free flow of water. Insert the tube into the rectum. The flow of water can be adjusted with the knob attached to the tube. When all the water has been introduced, remove the tube and resist the pressure for a few minutes. The bowels can be emptied after a while for better cleansing. If one does not wish to take enema in the lying position, he can take it in the standing position.

Enema can be given with benefit during fever, for constipation and almost in all diseases.

HOME REMEDIES FOR DIFFERENT SYMPTOMS OF IBS

Stomach Ache (abdominal pain)

☞ For immediate relief, powder one teaspoon of ajwain, curum and half teaspoon of jeera and mix in warm water.

To this add the juice of half a lemon and a pinch of rock salt and drink it at least twice a day.

- Mix 4 gm. *pudina* (spearmint), half teaspoon each of *saunf* (fennal seeds) and *ajwain* (curum) along with a pinch of rock salt and *hing* (asofoetida). Take it with warm water twice daily.
- Cut a lemon into half and add to it some rock salt, *kalajira* (black corawy) and pepper and suck it slowly.
- Boil four tender neem (Azadiracta) leaves in water, strain it and add two black peppercorns, a pinch of rock salt and drink twice a day.
- Dry and powder the outer skin of a pomegranate and eat half teaspoon of the powder with honey twice a day.
- Mix half a teaspoonful of the juice of *tulsi* (basil) leaves with one-fourth teaspoon of juice of ginger and drink with warm water.
- Mix one teaspoon of juice of jamun fruit (jumboline) with rock salt and drink it.
- Take a pinch of powdered *chotti harar* (Terminatia chebula) with warm water.
- Powder some mustard seeds and apply on the stomach for instant relief of pain and vomaiting.
- Drink half teaspoon of crushed garlic with warm water.

Foods to be avoided

- Fibrous fruits and vegetables.
- Spicy foods.
- Fatty foods.
- Meat, fish, etc.
- Pulses, beans and other pulses.

Indigestion

- Take one teaspoon of lemon juice, half teaspoon of crushed ginger, a small amount of *dhaniya* (Coriander leaves), *pudina*, one black pepper, a pinch of *jeera* and salt and grind it into a paste. Take this paste either half an hour before meals or immediately after meals.
- Take 200 gm. of *ajwain*, 4gm of *hing* and 20 gm of rock salt and powder them. Take 2 gm. of this powder twice a daily with warm water after meals.
- To one glass of fresh water, add juice of a medium sized lemon and drink it after every meal.
- Take half teaspoon each of juice of lemon and onion after each meal.
- Add roasted *jeera*, black pepper and salt to buttermilk and drink after meal.
- Add equal amounts of juice of ginger, lemon and orange and drink after each meal.
- Drink tomato juice to which rock salt is added, twice daily.
- To one teaspoon each of carrot juice and juice of *palak*, add two pinches of rock salt. Take this preparation early in the morning daily.
- Make a *chutney* of *pudina* leaves and add *hing*, *jeera*, black pepper, *ajwain* and salt. Eat this after every meal.
- Take a ripe papaya, cut it into small pieces and eat after adding salt, pepper and lemon juice.

Hyperacidity/Heart burn

- Drink coconut water daily to fight acidity.
- Take a few corinder leaves, crush and mix them in water. To this, add a pinch of rock salt and drink twice daily.
- Add two pinches of powdered *chotti harar* to honey and swallow twice daily.

- Mix one teaspoon juice of amla, one fourth teaspoon of roasted and powdered *jeera*, half teaspoon of powdered *dhania* and a small piece of *mishri* (sugar candy) and take it once daily after meals.
- Take a small amount of *palak* (spinach), five pieces of *parwal* and boil together. Add a few drops of juice of coriander leaves and salt. Cool this juice and drink twice daily. This improves the burning sensation and eructation.
- For acid eructation, take two teaspoon of juice of radish and add some mishri and take it twice daily.
- Chewing one clove after meals will reduce acidity.
- Drink one glass of shrerbet of *gulkand* twice daily.
- Take a few seeds of *bathua saag* and powder them. Take 2 gm of this powder with honey once daily. This keeps the bowel clean and removes excess acid.
- Take a few leaves of *peepul tree*. Dry and powder them. Take one teaspoon of this powder with water once daily.

Foods To be avoided

- Stale food.
- Spicy and oily food.
- Sweetmeats.

■

6

FOOD FOR DIGESTIVE SYSTEM

Mouth is the main doorway through which all our food enters into our stomach. From the stomach, process of digestion takes place in full form. As soon as the food enters into our mouth, it should be masticated and reduced to a fine pulp with the help of saliva. Such a well masticated food, when reaching the stomach, does not exert much strain on the stomach to overwork and exert much. Well digested food is the only source to energise, sustain and enliven various body functions. It is, therefore, well in order to eat only easily digestible food rich in all the essential vitamins minerals, green leafy vegetables, fats, carbohydrates, proteins etc. In a way one should always take a well balanced diet by which one's system should never be vitiated by unnatural means. Spicy, fried, fat rich, finely milled wheat flour and polished rice should always be avoided. Avoid all foods which are spice-rich and contain too much of saturated fats. As and when necessary, never miss an occasion for food substitutes lest your food becomes a cause for monotony. Use plenty of salads, fruit and vegetables juices, milk. Avoid condiments, red meats, all liquors, spices and condiments, fast foods etc.

■

7

COMMON DIGESTIVE DISORDERS

In this chapter some common digestive disorders are described for the benefit of readers.

CONSTIPATION

Impaction of bowels, weak peristaltic action of intestines, rectum and anus, dry and fatless foods, absence/lack of green and leafy vegetable, fruits, milk, absence of bulk forming agents may lead to constipation which is only a symptom and not a disease. Constipation is the biggest monster that triggers most of alimentary disorders. If you have constipation, you may suffer from:

- ☞ Flatulence and wind accumulation
- ☞ Pain in abdomen (Colic)
- ☞ Dysentery
- ☞ Blind or bleeding piles
- ☞ Hernia, strangulation
- ☞ Fistula, Fissures, Cancer of rectum/Anus etc.
- ☞ Acidity and heart-burn
- ☞ Sour and/or acidic eructations
- ☞ Pain in navel region
- ☞ Nausea, vomiting
- ☞ Headache
- ☞ General malaise and feeling of 'Not being well' or 'something is wrong with digestive organs and digestion.

Causes of Constipation

- ☞ Use of purgatives, habitually
- ☞ Absence of stool for many days, resulting in hard knotty and dry stools which are difficult to expel.
- ☞ Lack/absence of bran, leafy and green vegetables, milk, fruits
- ☞ Ingestion of junk food, fast food, highly spicy, fried and condimented foods
- ☞ Lack of physical activity
- ☞ Too much rest or activity
- ☞ Habitual and excessive use of alcohol, tobacco, narcotics etc.

Prevention

Avoid the factors listed above and also change life-style, way of thinking, working and approach.

DIARRHOEA

It is characterised by loose or semi solid stools, with or without abdominal pain. Real danger surfaces when too much of water and salts are lost to our body, resulting in general malaise, extreme thirst, unrest, griping pains, tenesmus, rectal pain and urgent urge to rush to the closet or, in some cases, watery stools escape in the clothes. Dehydration may cause, nausea and vomiting which are serious symptoms which might push a patient into comatose.

Infantile diarrhoea is a serious manifestation which is a known killer of infants and children.

Types

- ☞ Diarrhoea of infants and children
- ☞ Diarrhoea of young persons

- Diarrhoea of Travellers
- Diarrhoea of pregnant, post-natal ladies
- Senile diarrhoea (of old and aged people)
- Diarrhoea of drunkards, indolent, sedentary, glutt
- Diarrhoea due to dietary indiscretions
- Diarrhoea caused by anxiety, fear, apprehension, tension
- Summer Diarrhoea
- Diarrhoea of rainy/wet seasons
- Diarrhoea due to feasts, marriage dinners, club parties, social gatherings
- Beer Diarrhoea, etc.

If you look at the types of this malady, you will, at once, be able to discern and locate the cause that has triggered the malady. Once the underlying and precipitatory cause has been discerned, treatment is quite possible but the proviso remains that the patient must avoid and scruplously stay away from the causative factors. It is no using taking medicines every now and thereafter indulge in forbidden/harmful situations/foods. Prevention and corrective approach are the watchwords.

There is a causative and underlying factor that causes loose motions. Some preemptive and corrective steps must be taken before starting on a journey, before onset of seasons, when ailment returns or is anticipated to stage a comeback. Once you have corrected and modified your dietary means, most of diarrhoea related problems shall get relegated to the back seat. Chronic diarrhoea is a serious disease which requires thorough clinical investigations.

Do's

- Take rice, rice water, coconut water, lime water in plenty.
- Take 'Electral powder' to ward off danger of dehydration, water-sodium imbalance, thirst.

- Moong, rice and curd should be taken as meals.
- Drink boiled water only.
- Take light tea in moderate quantity.

Don'ts

- Eliminate fats, oil, dry fruits, milk and milk products, sauces, jams, chutnies, pickles etc.
- Refrain from spices and condiments.
- Do not consume junk/fast foods, so-called 'Office lunch', chats, juices sold in the bazars, cane sugar or any other cold drinks etc.
- Avoid strong tea, coffea, cocoa, wine, whisky, beer, tobacco, meats, fish etc.
- Don't be panicky and hasty and wait for the medicine to act.
- Don't jump from medicine or system to another in a hush, and do not use medicines of divergent therapies concurrently, due to drug interaction and drug reaction.
- Do not return to your normal dietary pattern immediately after you recover—allow some cushion time between recovery period and normalcy.

DYSENTERY

It is also a form of diarrhoea but, here, the stools are accompanied by mucus or blood or both which points to infection in the intestines. There is much pain, tenesmus, passage of mucus and blood tinged loose or semi solid stools. There is indigestion, bleeding, loss of weight, anaemia. The infection is brought on by food impurities resulting in ulceration of intestines and the occasional formation of abscesses in the liver. Amoebic dysentery is controlled by drugs like emetine and tetracyclines, but treatment has to be continued for a fairly long period—depending on severity and depth of infection.

Ameobic dysentery is generally confined to tropical and subtropical regions/countries.

Dysentery is a recurring phenomenon and auxilliary measures like intake of boiled water, cleaned and washed vegetables and fruits, high standard of personal hygiene. Ameobic dysentery is caused by a parasite or protozoan called Eantamaeba hystolytica.

Another type of dysentery is 'Bacillary Dysentery' which is caused and spread by bacteria of the genus 'Shigellia' and is spread by contact with a patient/carrier or through food, contaminated water or by faeces. This condition may spread in the form of epidemics. Infections include diarrhoea, fever, cramps, and they persist for a week or so. There could also be present dehydration and bleeding from the gut. Use of antibiotics efficiently controls the malady but may reappear if causes surface again.

Fluid and sodium losses should be controlled by 'Electral Powder' which should be taken in place of ordinary water. But, in any case, boil the water very thoroughly, in addition to taking safeguards, diet and hygienic measures suggested under this heading and diarrhoea. If vomiting and nausea also accompany dysentery, position becomes more serious and may assume form of cholera. In any case, accord topmost priority to control of bleeding and vomiting.

NAUSEA AND VOMITING

Feeling that one is about to vomit is called 'nausea' and is most common during travelling, seasickness, pregnancy (in early stage). The substance of food, bile, phlegm/mucus, water/ liquids purged out, subsequent to nauseatic feeling, and no vomiting which can also occur due to acidity, water brash, cholera, disagreeable food, odour of gases and chemicals, seeing some unpalatable event/scene or even seeing another person vomiting, nauseating filth and foul smell; high blood, pressure and headache (in some cases it is relieved by vomiting). Vomiting during 1st trimester of pregnancy is quite common and not unnatural but if it occurs on/after 7th month and the bouts are shattering and convulsing, an abortion may take place.

Vomiting and nausea can also be triggered by ingestion of drug, during/after operation, food poisoning (Ptomaine Poisoning), cold, cough etc. Certain causatives are beyond control but some can be offset by taking proper precaution and safeguards. Profuse and persistent vomiting is a serious and life threatening situation, when the patient should be put on saline-glucose drip into which some anti-emetic and anti nausea agents should be injected so as to restore saline-glucose and water level in the body and also for treating nausea and vomiting with requisite medicines.

Harrison has given following details about vomiting, "Vomiting is the reflex action of ejecting the contents of the stomach through the mouth. Vomiting is controlled by a special center in the brain that may be stimulated by drugs (e.g. 'Apomorphine') acting directly on it, or by impulses transmitted through nervous pathways either from the stomach (e.g. after ingesting substances and in stomach disorders), the intestine (e.g., in intestinal obstruction), or from the inner ear in motion sickness. The stimulated vomiting center sets off a chain of nerve impulses producing co-ordinated contractions of the diaphragm and abdominal muscles, relaxation of the muscle at the entrance to the stomach etc, casuing the stomach contents to be expelled." Vomiting is also called 'Emesis' in medical parlance.

Instead of going into the unnecessary details about causes, try to control vomiting and/or tone down frequency, restore sodium-water-sugar balance in the body, maintaining general resistance and strength of the patient. If situation is too grave to be controlled at home, rush the patient to doctor or call in the doctor. Remember, even a slight delay can prove fatal or, at least, complicate the case.

FLATULENT COLIC/GAS/WIND

When too much of wind producing eatables are ingested but the food remains stuck up in intestines, it gives rise to accumulation of gas/wind in the stomach, due to which the abdomen bloates and there is a gurgling sound. In majority of cases, there is also pain, restivity, sweating, uneasiness, unfructuous desire to visit the closet to pass stools-when neither stool nor wind gets expelled. I have taken up all the factors together because there is hardly any difference in symptoms, causes and complaints. The fact of the matter is that winds gets locked up, abdomen bloates, wind/gas does not pass and if such a situation lasts longer, there may be pain (colic) in the abdomen.

The root cause of all such disorders is overeating but, in other cases, when food is not taken for a longer period, even then there is accumulation of wind which, if not expelled, causes pain. The latter variety of colic yields when food is eaten in moderate quantity. The next cause of such complaints is constipation but all the symptoms subside as soon as stools are passed and wind gets discharged. If the pain lasts even after passage of wind and stools, it must not be taken lightly and got treated by a doctor. All said and done, all pains in the abdomen must not always be attributed to constipation and locking up of wind.

Colic is rather a confusing term which is also called for Renal colic, Intestinal colic, Billiary colic, Gallstone colic, Flatulent colic, etc. The name of the disorder points to the involvement of a particular organ being at fault. Hence, when treating a case of colic, always try to find out which of the organs in alimentary tract is at fault—once the organic cause has been properly discerned, there is not likely to be any difficulty in treating the agonizing disease and its symptoms.

If wind fails to pass through downwards, it may travel upwards and, thus, exert pressure on the heart region which is misconstrued as Angina pectoris (pain in the heart region) but symptoms are so variable in both the conditions that there is hardly any distinction between the symptoms.

ACIDITY AND HEARTBURN

These conditions point to depraved digestive system for which so many factors are accountable. Even a small deviation, late lunch or dinner, overeating, consumption of liquor, tobacco, spices, fats, excess of meats and fish, high protein but low carbohydrate diet, recent or chronic constipation or sedentary habits.

Symptoms

Frequent heartburn and acidity can adversely affect liver, stomach and its lining, enzyme production and, above all, entire digestive system is thrown out of gear. There is a constant burning sensation, acidic/sour eructations, restivity, pain or discomfort. Usually character of pain is of burning which is felt behind the breastbone and often appears to rise from the upper mid abdomen, either towards or into the throat. The patient feels as if the ingested food would come upto the mouth and that he may have to vomit but vomiting doesn't, generally, occurs. Heartburn might be accompanied by appearance of bitter or acidic fluid in the mouth, and is generally and quite often caused by regurgitation of the stomach contents into the gullet or by esophagus.

If there is nausea and much restivity, at once precipitate vomiting which will relieve and mollify most of the symptoms but bitter and acidic taste will be left in the throat and mouth.

PEPTIC ULCER OR ULCER OF STOMACH

Excess of acids is the major factor that causes sour eructations, stomach upset and indigestion or heartburn and we try to mollify such symptoms by taking antacids which are considered to rectify and prevent sour eructations. Infact, hydrochloric acid is a natural constituent of stomach secretions, and helps the digestive enzymes to activate. Recurrent bouts of excessive acidity permeate in the form of peptic ulcer which is a condition of localised destruction of mucosa of stomach or inner wall of the stomach (gastric ulcer). When upper part of small intestine gets infected, it gives rise to duodenal ulcer, or we can say that it is a wound inside the stomach or duodenum. Persons, who have 6 to 8 times more acid than is normally required, do suffer from peptic ulcers but there are many exceptions also, hence this is not a standard criterion. There are cases which have low grade acidity but, even then, they have peptic ulcers.

Excessive use of spices, condiments, alcohol, tobacco, coffee, tea etc. Can be the basic cause of peptic ulcer. In addition, there are drug-induced peptic ulcers which are caused by indiscreet/overuse of resperine, caffeine, corticosteroids, indomethacin, brufen, aspirin etc.

Symptoms

- Pain in upper part of the abdominal region, usually aggravated by food.
- Pain is sharp, penetrating and of burning type.
- In gastric ulcers pain increases soon after or immediately after taking meals but, in case of duodenal ulcers, it (pain) may occur 2-3 hours after taking meals. These are variable timings of occurrence which clearly distinguish pain, in one ulcer from another.

Type of ulcer can be finally determined after barium renal test, examination of stomach and its contents.

The problem can complicate when there is bleeding/ perforation at the site of ulcer, in that case surgery becomes necessary but, in all other situations, specified drugs and general measures will resolve the problem.

Generally cold and toned milk nullifies the problem but a bland diet also solves the problem. Milk may be served to the patient small quantities of milk can be taken frequently say every minutes on even 2 hours, depending on severity/intensity of the case. Milk counteracts acidity and also delays emptying stomach, thus allowing the drug to act for much longer period.

JAUNDICE

In healthy state, bile is expelled into the duodenum during the process of digestion and is absorbed again. But, when excess of bile circulates in the blood, it gives rise to yellow colour (tint) in the eyes, nails, skin, renders urine deep yellow in colour, with passage of white stools. Prominent symptoms of jaundice are bitter taste in the mouth, slow pulse, extreme debility and exhaustion, either diarrhoea or constipation, pain in liver region.

CIRRHOSIS OF LIVER

Also called interstitial hepatitis, nutmeg liver or sclerosis of liver. Generally a chronic condition of the liver with an increase in the connective tissue but decrease in its size, alongwith degeneration of the parenchyma.

Alcohol is the chief factor. Next cause is carrying away of irritants to the liver by the blood vessels or by way of the capsule. Drugs like Arsenic, Quinine, Phosphorus, improperly made food, food poisoning, infectious diseases, syphilis, and obstruction of the bile ducts.

Symptoms

- ☞ Anorexia (loss of appetite)
- ☞ Nausea, with/without vomiting
- ☞ Bad taste and belching
- ☞ Pressure in epigastriurn
- ☞ Tenderness in region of liver
- ☞ Hepatic colic
- ☞ Breathlessness
- ☞ Occasional full red tongue
- ☞ Jaundice of skin
- ☞ Occasional constipation

- Enlargement of liver
- Skin looks dirty, of mudy colour
- Bleeding from gastro-intestinal passage
- Oedema beneath the eyes, genitals, legs and feet.
- Urine is high-coloured, heavily loaded with urea, some amount of bile but albumin and casts may also appear in the urine when kidneys are also involved.
- Temperature is usually normal or below normal but in some cases may elevate to 101°F or slightly higher (in rare cases).

Alcoholism/Syphilis are considered to be the precipitatory factors. As a rule cirrhosis of liver is almost incurable but further damage might halted if diagnosed and treated at the initial stage. With proper dietary regimen, safeguards, and by giving up alcohol totally may prove productive, or at least arrest further progress of the malady.

HEPATITIS

This must not be confused with jaundice or any other depraved liver function or disorder. Here, some virus infection causes inflammation of the liver or amoebic dysentery and lupus. Infectitious hepatitis is generally caused by contaminated food or drink, either by a patient or a carrier and generally occurs where there is poor sanitation.

Symptoms

After an incubation of 15-30 days the patient develops fever and nausea, yellow discolouration of the skin (as in jaundice) appears after a week or so thereafter, and persists for about 3 weeks. There are not much complications as the disease generally yields to treatment and doesn't recurr, except when the patient gets again infected. In any case, proper treatment can provide immunity.

Treatment : Injection of 'Gamma Globulin' provides temporary protection.

Hepatitis-B

This generally occurs in drug addicts. The infection is transmitted by blood or blood products that contaminate injection needles. That is the reason why disposable syringes and needles are recommended to be used when an injection is intended to be given. There is hardly any chance of infection when disposal syringes are destroyed after being used once only. In some places, those used syringes are not destroyed and, thus, used for other patients. This is unethical and condemnable practice. So, whenever you are to be injected always carry your own syringe and needle and destroy the same after taking the injection. Treatment depends on the type of infection.

Symptoms

Headache, fever, chills, jaundice and general weakness. The disease can be identified by detection of 'Australian Antigen' in the blood.

WORMS

There is hardly any person (of any age or sex) who had never had worm infestations, rather it would be more correct to say that alomost every person carries worms in the intestines. This is a major public health problem and the number of infected persons is on the rise. Worm infection is present to the extent of 90 percent in the residents of tropical countries, like India where standard of personal and general hygiene is apallingly low and the underlying cause is an impure and contaminated water supply, unhealthy environments, and socio-economic status. The position is worse in other Asian and African countries where hygiene standards are poorer.

Generally an infected person doesn't know about presence of worms unless there are serious complications and problems. Once eradicated, through medication, the worms hatch and cause agonizing distresses again, so, a total immunity from worms cannot be had, due to recurrence factors. Lack of knowledge, as to hygiene, water and vegetables contamination and impurities, prohibitive and high cost of medicines which not many people can afford, lack/absence of proper medical facilities (more so in remote corners and villages, small towns) and high rate of infection are some of the contributory factors that lead to various worms and worm-related disorders—some of which are quite serious and may threaten even life.

Types of Worms

- Roundworms
- Hookworms
- Pinworms
- Tapeworms
- Threadworms
- Giardia
- Whipworms

It may be remembered that worms hatch only where there is filth and filth is created by chronic constipation when stools remain lodged in the intestines and cannot be compelled due to weak/absent peristaltic action of intestines and rectum. In fact faeces remain lodged in the intestines for days together and putrify there, giving birth to various types of worms, constipation, foul smell, gas formation, flatulence, gastralgia etc.

As long as worms remain lodged in the intestines there are symptoms like gnashing of teeth, pillow wetting, irritation in the anus, occasional pain, general distress in abdomen, incarcerated and foul smelling wind, constipation, occasional piles (blind or bleeding) etc. Problem gets complicated and serious when worm infection travels to liver (as in the case of amoebic dysentery). Worms may even travel to brain or, for that matter, any other part of the body. But, once the body has been freed from worm infestations, most of the symptoms disappear and normal health is restored. If ever anyone or more of the said symptoms are felt or observed, get the stools tested which, in all probability, will disclose the type and presence of worms in the system. Once it has been confirmed as 'Positive', there should be no delay in treating the patient.

CANCER OF STOMACH

This is a dangerous disease but can be contained to some extent if detected at the initial stage. Sometimes even the patient also neglects this disease because symptoms are not that glaring or even disturbing but, when the actual malady is detected at later stage it is too difficult to cure.

Women children rarely suffer from stomach cancer.

Causes: Hot drinks, foods, hard fibre and injuries, alcohol, tobacco, drug addiction, irregular food habits, tension are some of the predisposing factors. Chronic state of peptic ulcers may also lead to cancer.

Symptoms: These are insidious in their development. It was previously thought that absence of HCL/Hydrochloric acid results in cancer, whereas excess of HCL surfaces in the form of ulcer. It is a fact that in the majority of cancerous cases there is no HCL. Prominent symptoms are listed below.

- ☞ Acidity and indigestion.
- ☞ Fetid breath, flatulency.
- ☞ Sensations could be either sharp or dull, burning, gnawing, sticking.
- ☞ Tenderness on touching or pressure applied over the painful region.
- ☞ Vomiting. If cancer is at the cardiac end of stomach, vomiting comes soon after, but if it at the pylorus (opening of stomach mouth into the intestines), vomiting comes several hours after taking food.
- ☞ Marked anaemia and general emaciation.
- ☞ Slow action of the heart, feeble pulse and rapid respiration

- Earthy or waxy colour of the skin.
- Edema of ankles.
- Pain radiates from stomach towards back or behind the shoulders.

PILES (HEMORRHOIDS)

Piles is found in two forms—when there is no bleeding but pain is severe and unbearable and whole rectum aches due to painful passage of hard, dry and knotty stools. Another form is of bleeding piles when there is much oozing of blood from the rectum and there are grape-like boils in and around the anus. The eruptions look like bunch of small grapes.

Causes

- Elimination of fats, milk and milk products from diet and too much consumption of dry food items.
- Irregular eating and working hours or else sedentary life style and lack of physical activity.
- Excessive use of alcohol, spiced food, tea, coffee, cocoa, tobacco, drugs etc.
- Habitual use of purgatives.

Symtpoms

Mentioned here are combined symptoms of both types of piles.

- Pain before, during or after stools and sometimes pain persists in all the three conditions.
- Enlarged and tangled, hard and swollen veins.
- Great tenesmus and constriction.
- Bleeding at the end of defecation.
- Inability to sit, move or even lie down.

Corrective measures

- Regulate food timings, rest and proper physical activity.
- Avoid using cushioned seats, synthetic canes, but use airy chairs where air can easily let in.
- Take plenty of milk, green and leafy vegetables, pulpy fruits, coconut water, radish, cane sugar juice.
- Eliminate spices, condiments, liquor, tobacco, purgatives.
- Take 1-2 teaspoon of Isapghul husk with lukewarm milk. Some pure ghee may also added but do not use any strong purgative.

■

8

NATUROPATHY—TO CURE DIGESTIVE DISORDERS

According to Naturopathy, food, wrong (food) eating habits, eating every time not giving rest to digestive organs, overloading stomach with frequent and unwanted food items, constipation lack or absence of sweating, interrupted urinary flow, vitiation of three humours, improper and inadequate rest or dietary habits, use of health damaging items like alcohol, tobacco, tea, coffee, intoxicants and drugs, excessive use of spicy, fatty, condiments foods. Unbalanced and nutritionless food etc. are the major causes of various types of disorders, out of which obesity and its offshoot disorders form major diseases.

Naturopathy aims at excretion of toxins and waste matters from our body through fasting, enema, by inducing perspiration, regulating bowels and urinary flow. Even Ayurveda subscribes to all the said methods when it gives efficacy of fasting, purging, catharsis, purification (Shodhan), sweating (Swedana) etc. All such devices are supplementary to the leading curative method, by whichever name we may call it.

Since our main subject is obesity, I will confine myself only to the methods which help to purge the body, normalises breathing and circulatory and cardiac efficiency, promotes and facilitates free flow of urine, expulsion of faecial matter (stools), induce sweating, keep up mobility of limbs and, above, all general maintenance of health. Following methods/techniques are generally applied to gain the aforesaid advantages , viz.:

1. Enema
2. Hip Bath

3. Sun-Bath
4. Fasting
5. Massage
6. Fruit and vegetable therapy
7. Hot foot-bath
8. Steam-bath

ENEMA

Spread a sheet on floor and lie on a hard surface, ensuring that your body touches the floor except hips, which should remain slightly elevated. Use a utensil which should hang down from a wall. Clear the tube, nozzle and utensil and let out some drops of water from the nozzle so that no air remains trapped therein. It will rule out possibility of air-pocket which shouldn't spill over to intestines and stomach. Now insert the nozzle into the rectum to facilitate free entry of water. When it is felt that requisite quantity of tepid water has entered the intestines, close and remove the nozzle and wait until pressure and urgency to defecate. Visit the closet when you feel it is no more possible to hold on water in the intestines. You may hear rumbling or gurgling sound of water in the stomach. Initially it may take some time to create urgency/desire for defecating but, when your intestines get used to enema water, such an urgency can surface earlier, with passage of time. To begin with, first of all water will gush out followed by stools of pasty or loose consistency. When you have emptied your bowels, give some rest to your body. In some cases one may have to visit the closet more than once which is quite natural and need not cause and upset or worry.

Persons, suffering from habitual constipation, may add ½ to 1 teaspoon of castor oil to water but no salt should be used. Enema must not be taken daily, but may be taken after 7-10 days, as daily enema use will make the intestines dependent thereof and one won't be able to pass stools without taking an enema. Those who are suffering from diarrhoea or dysentery must not take enema. Enema facilitates smooth passage of stools, doesn't let hard stools form, removes even chronic constipation, improves peristaltic action of bowels (intestines, rectum and anus). Enema must not be followed by fasting but one can take only light diet and some seasonal fruits and salads in moderate quantity. Avoid and resist the temptation of fried foods, fats, species, condiment, meat, fish or alcohol. Take only bland and easily digestible diet.

SUN-BATH

Had there been no sun, there wouldn't have been any growth of vegetation, water wouldn't have flown down from the snow clad mountains, seasonal changes would have become a daydream. Infect sun protects, nurtures, develops, feeds, controls our various activities. Sunrise heralds advent of day and sunset indicates impending arrival of night. Sun-bath is a natural source of vitamin-D. It induces perspiration, thereby helping the toxins to excrete from our body, through skin pores. It also imparts much needed energy to our body. Infact life wouldn't have been possible without sun.

Sun-bath is possible during winter days when natural heat is required by the body to sustain itself. In some rural areas people keep tepid water (stored in a bucket or some other utensil) under sun for 1-2 hours and then bathe naked/semi-naked in the sun. It has multifold advantages - Sun rays fortify medicinal properties of water, keep it lukewarmed, solar energy (which consists of seven colours) reaches even minutest parts of our body and there is no fear of exposure. If whole body is massaged under direct sunlight/ rays, oil will reach easily within our body, providing it a renewed energy and vigour. Further, all the skin pores will open and sweat glands get energised, sweating process will be activated so as to excrete toxins through skin pores.

Sun-bath has inherent therapeutic values, but in the west it is used as a cosmetic device only. In more sensitive persons sun-bath is not advised due to chance of exposure to cold, nor should they massage or take bath in the open. However, such persons should fully wrap up their bodies with a blanket if, at all, they are keen to have a sun-bath.

FASTING

It is a gateway to bliss and health. It not only purifies the body, it also purifies the mind. In a way, it tones up, fortifies, purifies and sublimates body and mind. It takes away animal insights and inculcates higher values and laudable habits. To say that fasting is simply a way to starve the body is merely an attempt to underestimate it. Its importance lies in the fact that most, if not all, of the holy books laid stress on fasting and rightly recognised it as a gateway to heaven. Fast should never be implied to mean that it is simply a way to abstain from food rather to set in order all imprudent use of foods, besides removing acidity, gas, and flatulence. It corrects and tones up entire digestive system. In fasting, balance in body juices is moderated, improved, various mechanisms that produce blood, bones and flesh are totally corrected/overhauled, and cleansed, chemical balances brought under normal functioning. It also is a great purger of toxic elements, a great cleanser of filth, normalisers and restorer of health, renders body agile and light. Moreover, our tired and overtaxed body and organs do get a well deserved rest. During the first two or three days, there may be felt some uneasiness, but regular practice will take away such element(s). It is said that—

> "Whosoever fasts is blessed in every way as he draws the benefit of great medicines. All the diseases are cured and he becomes strong and virile".

Who should not Fast

Following categories of persons should abstain from fasting process.

1. Pregnant and confined mothers before, during and after delivery and, more particularly, who are anaemic, emaciated, and run-down and can't afford well balanced and nutritious food.

2. Mothers who are breast-feeding their infants.
3. Persons suffering from T.B., epilepsy, ulcers, labourers doing arduous manual work.
4. Persons during the course of actual travelling.
5. Old persons who are bed-ridden, unable to move, have stiff and immobile organs and eat far less than their actual requirement—in a way, the under and malnourished ones.
6. Weak, emaciated and starved children who are in their growth stage and also ladies belonging to that category.
7. Those who utilise fasting as a ploy for overating and who indulge in dietary indiscretions.
8. Persons suffering from low blood pressure and low sugar levels in their blood.

Who should take to Fasting

All the classes and conditions which are prohibited to fasting process, described earlier, can resort to fasting who satisfy the reverse of described conditions and health state. Following persons must take to fasting either completely, for the whole week, on all alternate days or, at least once week or fortnight, depending upon necessity and urgency.

1. Persons who often overeat, are gluttons and always continue to eat one eatable or the other.
2. Whose bowels are either impacted or often get loose motions.
3. Who suffer from dysentery, diarrhoea, colic, locking up of gas, rigidity of joints and other limbs.
4. Diabetics whose blood sugar level is generally high.
5. Habitual drunkards of alcoholic drinks, smokers, fast food eaters, obese and sedentary persons who eat too much but shun physical activity.
6. Children who are easy-going, relish foods prepared outside their homes.

What to do during Fasting

1. Mix a teaspoon each of lemon juice and honey in 150 ml water (cold or lukewarm) early in the morning and drink it. It will provide energy to the body. The same preparation may be repeated in the afternoon or some non-irritant liquid instead.
2. Do not remain stuck to chair or bed but attend to your daily chores, including physical activity.
3. Except when medically advised/necessitated, no medicine should be taken during fasting—not even well exhorted tonics. Let the our physician be your guide in this respect, as far as use of medicine is concerned.
4. Fasting does not protract divorce from diet or any ingestion of food. Even while on fasts, you are allowed to take permissible eatable/drinks.
5. During summer season never starve your body from water which is our life force. There is no harm in taking a glass of orange or lemon juice which will help to purge our toxic, facial and unwanted matters from the body but will also strengthen the body.
6. No toxic food should be taken during fasting.
7. Fasting must not be utilised as an occasion and excuse for consuming fat-enriched, alcoholic, spicy, meat-based preparations or any other eatable which you have been forbidden.
8. If one wishes, one can resort to partial fasting for a week, each day you exclude one or two of these items viz. salt, sugar, grains, fats, spices, certain fruit or/and vegetable milk products. This way your body will have an almost disease free menu, when certain excess and shortages would be fully balanced. But a complete fast, at least once a fortnight or month, is also all the more a necessity. When you exclude one or more items, you will yourself come to realise what item harms or benefits you and such a discerned conclusion should serve you as a guideline, enabling you to draw a long lasting food regimen.

9. Avoid alcohol and tobacco, drug and toxins, at least during the course of fasting.
10. Due care must be given to health status, age, sex, weight, work schedule and its demands on your energy expense. If you ignore such and any other viable factors, you will only expose yourself to problems which may lead you in a position of 'No-Return'.
11. Not taking anything during fasting or else overating are the two extremes which should never be allowed to surface. Stick to what suits or does not suit you, instead of harping on what others say or eulogise or what is written in the books. It is reiterated that other experience may be your nightmare or vice versa. It is your own body, and none else could take care of it as you can, as you only know what is good or bad for you. You can always take a cue or inspiration from other person's personal experience and opinions but such averments cannot, and must not, be generalised. So, try to tailor all methods, opinions and suggestions to your own needs, depending on your own limitations, and compulsions. In short, try to be your own master. Listen to, what others say or preach, but never succumb to temptations, avoid indiscretions and imprudent conclusions.

Fast, if stretched beyond your sustainable capacity, can be more harmful than 'no-fasting' approach.

FOOD

To keep your body in good humour, food is the most important factor. Truly speaking, 'we are what we eat' or ' our food habits mould our mental faculties also'. You can live without water for a few hours, without air for some moments and without food also you can survive, but merely survive. When body is not nurtured and nourished with suitable foods, our body gives in, giving way to many health problems. If your body is not in a healthy state, mind also has to bear the brunt thereof, because a healthy mind lives in a healthy body. A lot has been written and spoken about food, proper food, food fads, fast foods, prohibited and acceptable and suitable foods. But, the fact remains that all foods do not and cannot suit all human beings as food allergies and reactions have a lengthy list of disorders. Naturopathy believes that most of our disorders stem from our wrong food habits and, vegetable and non-vegetable and non-vegetable diets, are both the culprits in this respect.

Following points on food intake may be of help to the readers (With particular reference to fasting under naturopahtic norms).

1. Take foods what suit you and, that too, at the punctual time. If you have skipped over a meal, there is no harm but overating or making up for the diet that you have missed is neither wise nor advisable.
2. Avoid all diets which abound in or contribute to formation of toxins, because once the body is ridden with poisonous elements, your entire energy would be expended in getting rid of them.
3. Avoid white sugar but the same may be substituted with jaggery and sugar-cane juice.
4. Water of tender coconut will help to mollify acidity, restore normally to impacted bowels.
5. Milk curd, cheese and whey also help the body to purge out toxins from the body and also serve as mild and gentle laxatives.
6. Milk, curd, cheese and whey also help the body to purge out toxins from the body and also serve as mild and gentle laxatives.
7. Any food taken should not retard and impede the process of elimination which includes excretion of urine, faeces, phlegm, wind and perspiration.

MASSAGE

Massage is a simple and effective method attain and maintain ideal health. Therapeutic massage has been a well known method (that still exists in various cultures and civilizations dating back to thousands of years) profusely and frequently employed to promote general well-being. Self esteem, to boost immune and circulatory systems, to normalise blood pressure, remove extra fat content from the body, regulate respiration, improve digestion, muscle tone and skin tone. Different massage techniques have been successfully employed, developed and integrated into various therapies.

In some countries 'Massage Parlours' are nothing other than prostitution centres but, of late, visit to such parlours is a status to symbol of the elite class. Even most of the modern 'health centres' are fully equipped and manned by massage experts.

Key Principles

1. Massage can rejuvenate and invigorate body.
2. It can aid in relaxation of tired and aching muscles and painful and stiff joints.
3. Creates a sense of general well being and comfort.
4. Takes away tension from mind.
5. Lowers the amount of circulating stress hormones.
6. Promotes elimination of chemical wastes from the body, such as lactic acid which is said to lead to pain and stiffness in joints and muscles.
7. Opens up pores of the skin so as to help in inducing perspiration.
8. Improves mobility and flexibility.

Basic Techniques: Mainly our techniques are employed for massaging viz. :

(*i*) Stroking (or Effeurage): When hands glide smoothly and rhythmically over the skin, either in a circular or slow fanning motion or alternatively.

(*ii*) Kneading: This action is like kneading a dough and hands are used alternatively to squeeze and release flesh rhythmically between the thumbs and fingers.

(*iii*) Friction: This method is employed for deep penetration, when even pressure is applied from the thumbs to a static point on the spine, or as small circles on the skin.

(*iv*) Hacking: Hacking is done with hands relaxed and working quickly over the skin. Here the side of the hands deliver alternate short, sharp taps on the body.

Vehicle used: Generally light vegetable oils or talcum powder is usually used as a vehicle for massage so that the hands glide over the skin. One may add essential oil to vegetable massage oil.

Precautions

- In case of any ailment, consult your doctor before embarking upon any non-conventional therapy.
- Do not massage during temperature rises, fractures, swellings, skin infections.
- Do not massage abdomen, legs and feet during first 3 months of pregnancy and, even after that, do not massage unless advised by a doctor.
- First, get lumps and swellings checked by a doctor.
- Cancer patients may get massage, only if medically advised, from a trained practitioner only.
- Stop blending essential oil with vegetable oil, if any unusual symptom or discomfort is felt. Better consult a physician. Highly sensitive skins may even react to ordinary vegetable oils.

How to proceed

Some other person should do massage for another person because only another person can perform this job more efficiently and effectively. There must be a gap of 1-2 hours between massage and food intake. Always get body massaged on empty stomach, after attending to calls of nature, but without taking bath. Use a wooden plank or spread a thick blanket on the floor. Apply mustard/olive/coconut oil over skin and apply pressure equivalent to 5 pounds on tender organs and 5-10 pound pressure over hands, feet, abdomen and chest, 15-20 pound pressure over organs above waistline, like back, upper part. Actual pressure will depend on a person's physical condition. Fat accumulates generally around waist, abdomen, legs and arms, hence these body parts must be massaged more thoroughly. Some people advise inserting a few drops of mustard oil in ears, nostrils, navel, rectum but medical acceptance of such device still remain unconfirmed.

Our body has two extremities in the form of hands and feet as all the nerves end here. If palms of hands soles of feet are thoroughly massaged, it will almost impart the benefits that are derived from accupresure method. Massage of palms and soles activates endocrine glands and all trigger points in the body, thus improving function of all the body organs.

Massage can be done from 15 to 60 minutes, depending paying capacity of the patient and also the involvement of affected organs. After massage has been finished, relax for an hour or so, but do not drink/eat anything until you finish bath which may be had after an hour of the massage. Use some glycerine soap to remove residues of oily substance. Body massage should be done in the morning, before sunrise in the morning in summer season and after 2-3 hours of sunrise in winter season. Use lukewarm water for bathing purposes in winter or tepid water in summer. During massage body sweats profusely and it is advised by experts that sweat should be re absorbed into the skin; hence not wiped. Sivanand advised that, in order to ensure quicker penetration and absorption of massage oil, it should be mixed with some amount of table salt and also that oil may be heated or lukewarmed before being massaged.

HYDROTHERAPY

Hydrotherapy is an integral part of Naturopathy (other facets having been described earlier) and cold bath, hot bath, steam bath, sitz bath, alternate hot and cold baths, whirlpool bath, compresses, Turkish bath, steam room baths or steam bath by sitting/standing in a cabinet, saunas and wraps are the major disciplines. This therapy is deemed to be a complete healing system by which an ailing body, overloaded with toxic and foreign matters, can be eradicated from the body through skin pores in the skin by sweat which is induced by hot/swim baths. This therapy is recognised both the conventional and non-conventional practice. Moreover, it is not new to India, Roman and Chinese who had been using it in one form or the other.

There is much evidence to prove that water has excellent ability to alter body's flow which could be manipulated varying its temperature, suiting an individual's capacity and health status. Cold water circulates blood to internal organs to enable them to reform their individual functions. It reduces BP., increases blood flow to skin, dilates blood vessels, thus easing stiffness also. It sends more nutrients and oxygen to the tissues, thus repairing the damage caused by various disorders. it also boosts immune system and improves blood circulation.

Mineral baths and mud have been known to allay tension, reduce circulatory congestion caused by spasm of muscles' and also are know to be beneficial in rheumatoid arthritis, better mobility and life of body joints. Some experts use cold and hot water alternatively.

Methods Employed

1. Sitz baths
2. Whirlpool baths
3. Hot or warm water baths.
4. Alternate hot and cold water baths.
5. Sea-water treatments.
6. Wraps
7. Compresses
8. Turkish baths, Steam Room and Steam Cabinets.
9. Saunas.

SITZ BATHS

Place two side by side-tubs/containers of water filling one with cold water and the other with hot water. The patient should sit for 3 minutes in hot water and one minute in cold water, keeping feet in the opposite bath. This position should be alternated.

Whirlpool baths

Immerse the body for 15 minutes in the pressurised bubbles and the body should be massaged.

Hot or warm water baths

Soak the body in hot water for 20-30 minutes, keeping temperature at 100⁰F or 38⁰C. If necessary oils, herbs and minerals can be added to warm bath. To derive better and quicker results, finely blended oatmeals/bran (couched in a muslin bag) to soothe skin, and minds, and extracts (such as Dead Sea salts) to nourish the skin or Epsom salts to relieve the swollen joints.

HOT FOOT BATH

Hot water should be used in winter and tepid water (if it is not too hot or cold) water in summer. Take a bucket wherein both feet can be immersed easily, and fill it to 3/4th capacity with suitable water adding, (if necessary), a teaspoonful of table salt. Now immerse both feet in the water, frequently massaging feet and legs in water itself. Keep the feet for about 20-30 minutes, and remove your feet from the water when it turns lukewarm. (In winter cover your body with a blanket so as to avoid exposure). If you have added salt to water, then pour hot water over your legs and feet after removing the same from water. Thereafter, wipe with a dry towel. After wiping take care that feet and legs are not exposed to cold winds.

Alternate cold and hot baths

Alternate hot and cold water therapies are credited with the benefits or stimulating hormonal system, reduce circulation related congestion (caused by muscle spasm) and relieving inflammation.

Sea Water Treatments

Sea-water is believed to possess healing properties while minerals inherent in seaweed are believed to induce sweating, tone and cleanse the skin. Seaside wraps, or sea water baths or sea-water itself, are also include in this system.

Wraps

In this process a cold flannel cloth-sheet is wrapped around the body and cold/hot packs are wrapped in towels for being placed on top. Then the patient is covered in a warm blanket and left for about 30 minutes. This process is employed to treat long-term fatigue, aid in circulation and to stimulate the immune system of patient.

Compress

Soak the towels in cold/hot water, wring out, and then apply to affected parts of the body so as to increase blood flow, make the body sweat and ease stiffness of muscles through hot compresses. Cold compresses are employed to reduce inflammation and push up circulation of blood.

Turkish baths, (steam) cabinets and steam rooms

If a patient sits in a steam room for about 20 minutes or for an hour in a cabinet, sweat will be induced, impurities eliminated and water relieved received. This procedure is known as Turkish baths.

Saunas

Though saunas are identical to Turkish baths they generate dry heat and not humid heat. For Sauna, hot and dry temperature is required (say 100^{0}F or 38^{0}C). It encourages sweating and helps the body to eliminate waste products and impurities. After every 5-10 minutes during the sauna and at the end of the sauna, a dip or plunge into pool or cold shower is advised.

Precautions about the said devices

- During 1st trimester of pregnancy avoid sitz or steam baths, and during the next 6 months of pregnancy do not have treatments which exceed duration of 10 minutes.
- Patients of high blood pressure, heart disease or angina must avoid steam baths, saunas and hot baths.
- If a patient is asthmatic, epileptic, has undergone an operation or has a history of thrombosis, he must avoid all types of steam treatments.
- If one has an open wound, no ingredients should be added to bath. Patient who are allergic to iodine must avoid seaweed.
- Always consult and act upon the advice and guidance of a Naturopathy/Hydrotherpaist before embarking upon any of the discipline stated above.

Obese persons should weight on a weighting scale daily, and thereafter every week to know that benefits have accured and also what still needs to be done. One should aim to lose about one kg of body weight after a week and weight loss must be steady and gradual and even sudden and abrupt. Certain health clubs claim to shed enormous amount of weight within a week and often employ harmful techniques and strict dietary regiment to achieve their target which is not only undesirable but a health hazard also. Do not be misled by tall claims made by such weight reducing centres which have a covetous eye over your money. They are not concerned how much health and well-being you will have to sacrifice.

It is simply a matter of suitability as to which of the weight reducing devices and techniques could match with your physical competence; hence use your judgement in this regard but do not be misled by persuasion, publicity, big claims. If you wish, you may try your hand at western herbalists, Chinese herbalism, Auricular Acupuncture, Hypnotherapy, Homoeopathy, ayurveda, Tibetan Medicine—to mention a few only.

■

9

YOGA—TO CURE DIFFERENT DIGESTIVE DISORDERS

Yogasanas are helpful in maintaining figure and reducing weight. Yoga is an ancient science developed in India and propagated all over the world. The yogic exercises are good to reduce weight.

Sarvangasana

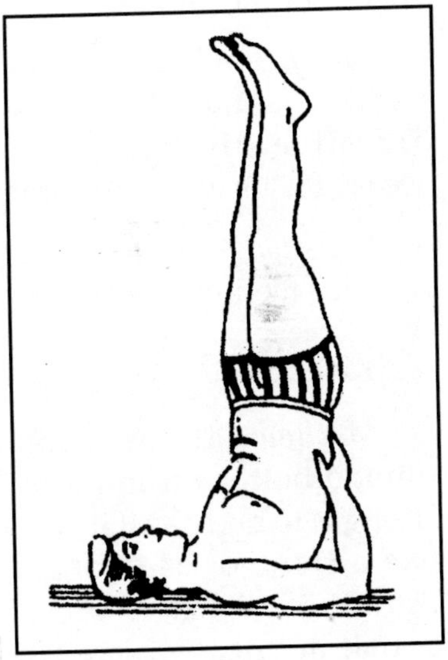

Method—Lie flat on the ground, your spine touching the floor, stretch the body, raise the legs slowly and let them stay at right angle to the trunk. After staying for a few seconds slowly raise up the body, without giving any jerk to the spine. Take help from the hands, keeping the fingers outward and thumbs towards the belly. Slowly go on raising the back until the whole trunk is at 90^0 and the entire weight comes on the shoulders and neck. Take the legs slightly forward and press the chest with your chin. After remaining in the said pose for a few seconds come to the original position.

Benefits—This asana cures constipation, dyspepsia, has a salutary effect on thyroid gland, tones up the nervous system, all limbs of the body, helps to preserve and thicken semen, is useful in intestinal disorders, varicose veins, appendicitis, renders spine flexible, throat disorders are removed, gas is expelled. In addition, it gives glow, vitality and strength to the body, increases sex power, removes menstrual disorders. Persons with hypertension and cordial problems should never take to this asana, except under advice and guidance and supervision of a yoga teacher.

Halasana

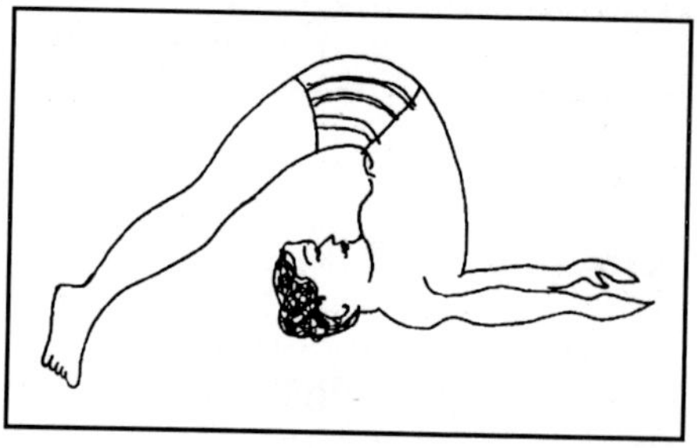

Method—Half of this asana is same as Sarvang-asana. Bend your legs behind your head and in doing this your head and knees should not bend.

Benefits—This is very good asana to cure digestive disorders and access fat on your abdomen.

Caustion—Try to bend your legs as much as you can bend without feeling any strain and slowly try to touch the ground.

Vajrasana

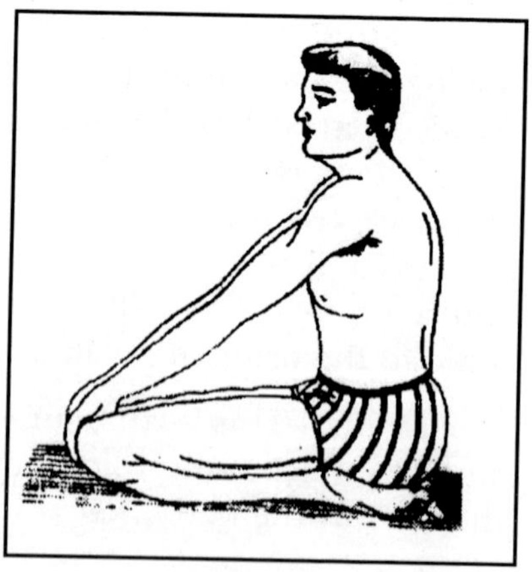

Method—It is named thunderbolt, as it imparts the strength to body as if it is made like a stone or as strong as a thunder bolt. It is the only asana, in yoga, which can be practised after 45 minutes or more from the time of finishing your meals. In between meal times, it can also be done, but never immediately after meals. Kneel down on the floor, letting your big toes, and legs and knees touch the ground. Now rest your buttocks on your knees, your heels bent inwards and thumbs touching each other. Place the palms on the knees, keeping your spine erect but relaxed and flexible. Breathing should be even, deep and slow. Expand your chest, drawing the abdominal muscles inwards.

Benefits —This asana will expel gas and remove acidity. How much you have overeating, it will digest the same. It tones up sexual system of both males and females, removes pain and stiffness in spine and knees, lowers raised blood pressure, gives longevity and retards and postpones old age. For meditation, it is an ideal asana, as you can sit in this asana for as long as you wish. After completion of this asana, simply massage with your hands or, still better, use salt mixed oil, say of mustard, which can be slightly lukewarm.

Bhujang or Sarpasana

Method—Lie flat on the ground, abdominal portion touching the ground. Straighten both the arms, palms touching the ground. Now bring the palms at level with both sides of abdomen. Slowly lift your neck and torso in such a way that whole body rests on your palms. Now lift your neck upwards gradually and try to look upwards as far and as conveniently you can. Let the toes touch the ground and palms securely

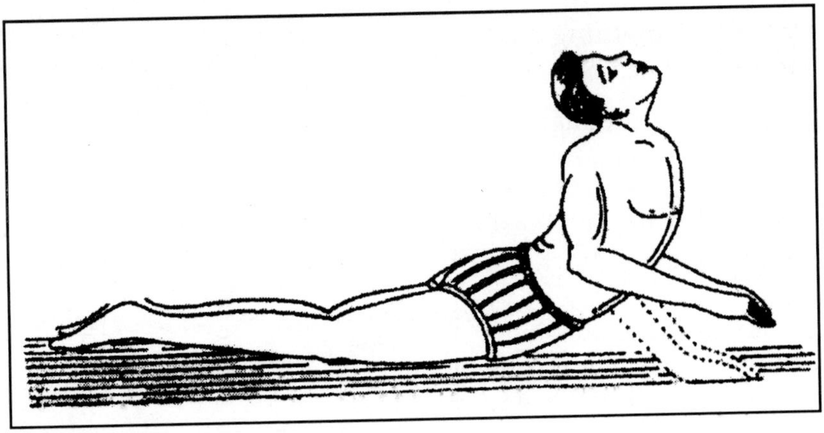

resting on the ground. Do not bend your elbows. Stay in the position as long you can. When you feel suffocated or when there is a feeling that you can't endure/continue any more, then slowly get back to original position from where you had started. After the asana is over, loosen your limbs and relax.

Benefits—Abdominal muscles and back portion are supplied with blood and blood circulation in general, is improved and also fresh and pure blood is supplied to all the organs. It imparts strength, flexibility and tone to spinal column. It removes menstrual disorders and irregularity, helps to improve digestion, chance of night discharge is dispelled, helps to maintain celibacy. It is useful for diabetics, as it activates the pancreas, thereby causing secretion of insulin, render arms, hands and neck painless, flexible and active. Kidneys and intestines are also to strengthened. It removes obesity, sheds extra flesh from the abdominal portion, and spinal curvature and postural abnormalities are also removed.

Chakrasana

Method—On a hard surface, lie flat on your back. Raise the middle portion of your body keeping both the feet and hands firmly on the ground thus making a semi-circle, ensuring that your head is kept between your hands. Now concentrate your eyes on something that lies in front of you.

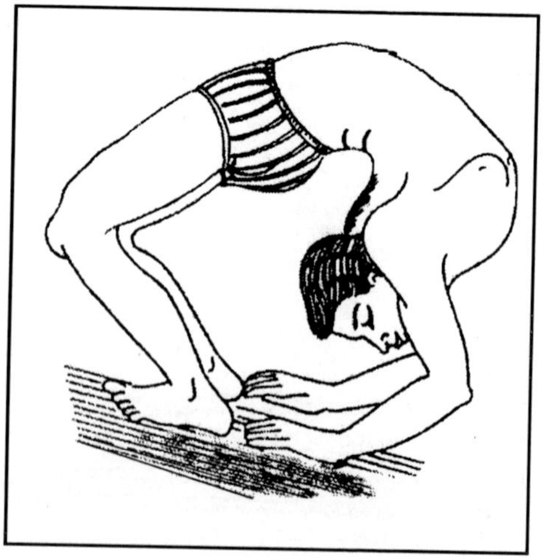

Benefits—It enhances, like the sarvanagasana, strength of head, throat, neck, abdomen, legs, hands and, in short, all parts of your body, eliminates pains in joints, removes extra fat from the abdominal area, activates digestive system, renders spinal column elastic and supple, imparts glow and agility to the body, normalises posture and stance, and the body stays erect even during the advanced age. Pregnant ladies should not practice this asana as it can adversely affect their pregnancy process even leading to miscarriage and bleeding.

Parvatasana

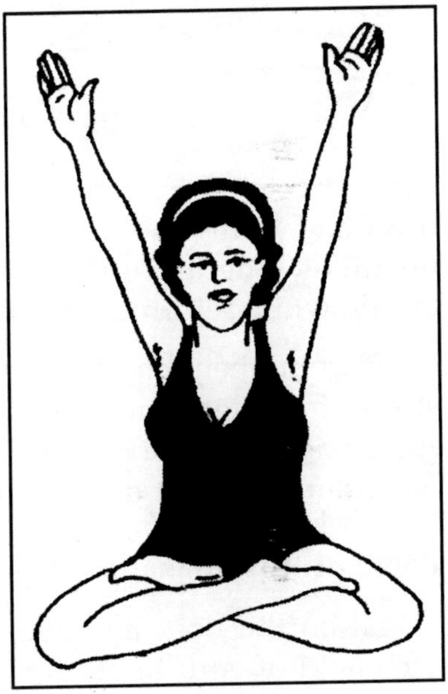

Sit in Padmasana (that is by keeping left foot on the right thigh and right foot on the left thigh). Inhale and raise both the hands towards the sky, keeping all the fingers apart and stretching both arms without bending. Stay in the said position as per your capacity and convenience but do not overdo. Gradually bring down both the arms and place on both the knees and relax, but without bending your back. Keep spinal column erect at 90°. The process can be repeated a number of times. In normal conditions ladies can also perform this asana, but never during pregnancy.

This asana imparts flexibility to the spine, strengthens arms, expands chest, and adds to strength of arms and fingers. Improves flexibility of shoulder blades. It improves upon asthmatic condition and tones up uterus.

Matsyasana

Sit in Padmasana and thereafter lie down on your back. Catch hold of big toe of feet with hands and rise up your back portion in a gradual manner. In this position your backside of

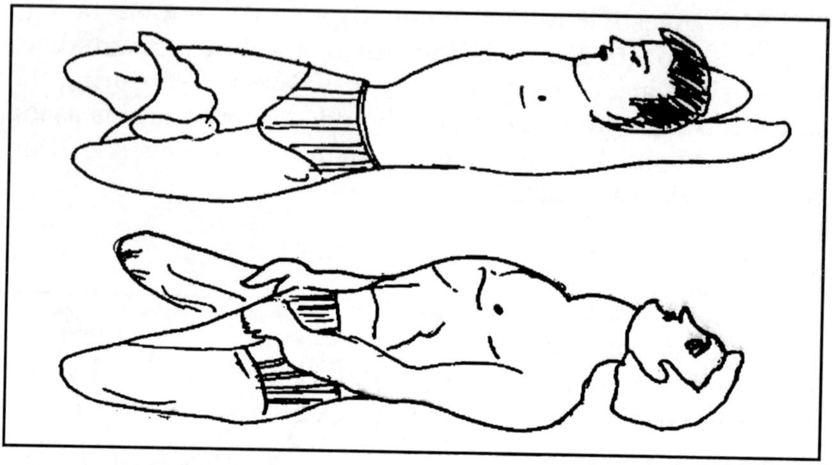

head and knees should continue to touch the ground. Retain breath as long as you can and stay in the final position and exhale while returning to the previous state.

It strengthens chest and lungs, removes extra fat from hips, strengthens legs and hands, dispels asthma, and removes constipation. In normal health conditions ladies can perform this asana, but not during pregnancy.

Pashchimottanasana

Sit on the floor and spread both legs in front of you and each hold of your big toes with both the hands, but do not let your knees bend. In order to catch the toes you have to bend the back. Initially it may seem slightly difficult to do so, due to rigidity of muscles and limbs; hence do not exert but gradually posture. In 4-5 sittings your body will get attuned to the final posture. Persons with

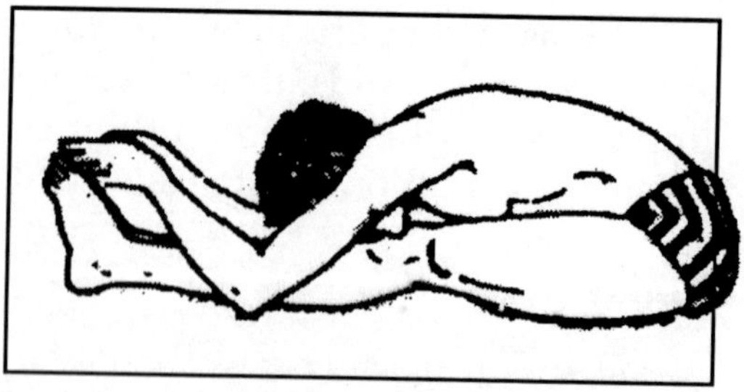

back pain and stiff and muscles, pregnant ladies should not perform this asana.

It strengthens legs, arms and renders the spine flexible and supple, improve digestion, removes fat on and around abdomen, constipation fortifies and rejuvenates energy and nervous system, lengthens leg bones, purifies blood, improves liver, cardiac and respiratory processes, removes fat from hips and sideways.

Those who get adept on this asana, may try to touch their knees with the nose but in the changed position knees shouldn't be bent.

Ardhamatsyendrasana

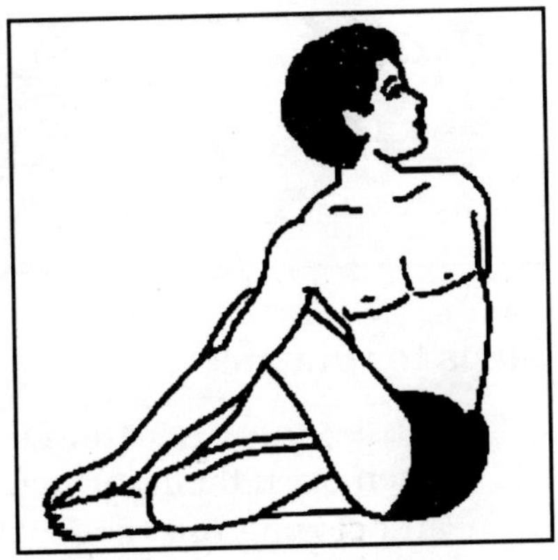

This exercise must be practised by almost every one because this asana and Vakrasana are the asanas that strengthen the spine in the vertical position. All other asanas performed lying on the back and abdomen bend the spine forward and backward. Doing Vakrasana first helps doing Ardhamatsyendrasana better and easily.

Method—Sit on the ground and place the left heel under the right thigh. Slowly take right leg across the folded left leg and place the foot flat on the ground near the left knee. Push the right leg pressing the abdomen by the left hand and place it touching the right foot or hold the right toes. Twist the waist towards right and bring your chin in level with your right shoulder. Take your right hand behind the back by twisting a little more and touch the right thigh. Stay for sometime in this posture and return to original position. Repeat the same with the other side.

Benefits—Useful for backache, digestive disorders, liver disorders, diabetes, kidney disorders and for obesity caused due to diabetes and indigestion.

Shavasana

Lie down on your back. Keep the whole body loose and in a straight position. Palms can be either on the floor or you can keep them upward. Do not use any pillow under your head. At this point keep breathing in normal way. Keep the eyes closed and let the whole body fall on the floor in an unrestrained way. This position should remain all through the actual practice.

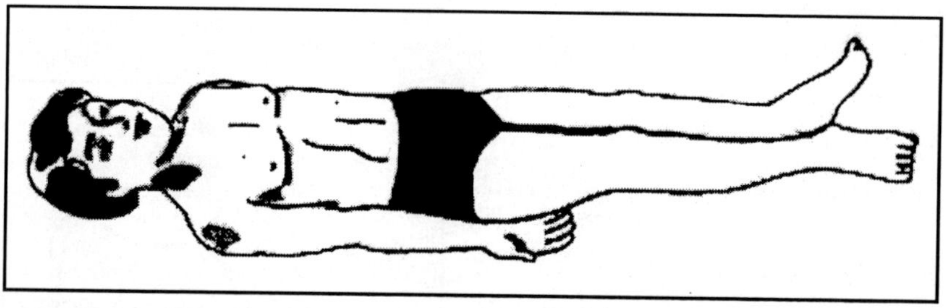

Steps for practice

- Close your eyes and keep them closed for two seconds. Then open them for two seconds. Do this simple opening and closing of eyes for three to four times.
- Open the eyes again and look upward, then downward then straight. Now look towards the left side, then towards the right side, then straight again and then close the eyes. Repeat this eye exercise two to three times.
- Now open your mouth wide without straining it. Turn the tongue inside the mouth in such a way that its tip is folded back towards the throat area, then close the mouth. Keep the mouth closed and tongue folded for 10 seconds. Then open the mouth and bring the tongue folded for 10 seconds. Then open the mouth and bring the tongue back to its normal position, then close the mouth. Repeat the process for two to three times.
- Keeping your eyes closed, bring your mental attention towards your toes. See (mentally) that the toes are

relaxed. Then move slowly upward and towards the head area mentally by checking the knees, thighs, waist, spinal cord, back, shoulders, neck, arms, palms, fingers and rest of the area of the body to be sure that they are actually relaxed. Make a slight movement of the neck and head by turning right and left. Then let the head rest at a comfortable position. Now the entire body is physically relaxed.

- *Then relax the mind with the following process:* Select a place of natural beauty which you have ever visited and liked, such as park, a garden, a lawn or a riverside and feel as if you are mentally present at that place. Attach your mind to that place. Feel as if you are lying at that place and breathing air of the same environment. Now while keeping the mind involved with that environment, do some deep breathing. In this deep breathing, just exhale and inhale slowly but deeply. During the breathing, the stomach should go upward while inhaling and it should come downward while exhaling. One exhalation and one inhalation make one round. Do not rush in this deep breathing. Make about ten to twelve rounds. When the deep breathing is over, feel as if you are going to sleep. Now relax completely. Stay in that position for 5 to 10 minutes. then open your eyes and stretch your body and then be seated. You have completed the Shavasana.

Benefits—Shavasana has a very good effect upon the doer. One immediate effect is that it relaxes all the muscles, nerves and the organs of the body. When the muscles, nerves and the organs are fully relaxed, they gain strength and their normal health is restored.

People suffering from insomnia, high and low blood pressure, gastric trouble, lungs and heart troubles and mental sickness, Shavasana is a remarkable kriya for providing immediate relief.

■

10

SIX YOGIC KRIYAS—TO CURE DIFFERENT DIGESTIVE DISORDERS

These Yogic Kriyas are the purification processes of the body by yogic methods. They are very important in Yoga. Union of body with mind, union of mind with soul and union of soul with God is Yoga.

Kriyas are to be practised early in the morning before sunrise on empty stomach. Kriyas must be finished before starting the Asanas or Pranayama.

These Kriyas consist of six purification practises:

1. Dhauti (Kunjal)
2. Basti
3. Neti
4. Tratak
5. Nauli, and
6. Kapalbhati.

Dhauti (Kunjal)

Washing stomach by water.

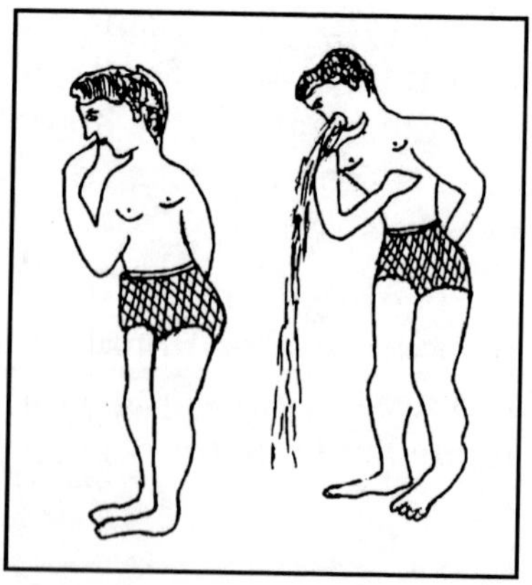

Two or three litre of tepid water is required. Squat on your feet your back, spine and neck should be straight. Drink glasses of tepid water continuously without any pause upto the brim of neck. One should neither talk nor laugh during this period. He should not bend and should stand.

Bend a bit forward. Keep the left hand on the left knee and the first and second finger of the right hand in your throat. Press the stomach by the other hand. You will vomit. Vomit the whole drunk water. Water should not remain in stomach.

Wash your hands and take rest. Milk or breakfast should be taken after an hour.

This Dhauti kriya should be practised after passing stool and after bath. One should not take bath after this kriya. Vaman Dhauti kriya should be practised once a fortnight or once a month.

Precautions

- Heart patients should not practise it.
- The nails of the fingers should be trimmed otherwise they may wound the throat.

Benefits

- Disorders of bile and gas are cured.
- It is beneficial in the diseases of stomach throat and jaundice.

Basti (Enema)

Enema pot, rubber tube, nozzle, tepid water, lemon are the requirements. Mix juice of one or two lemons in the tepid water. Fill the enema pot with water.

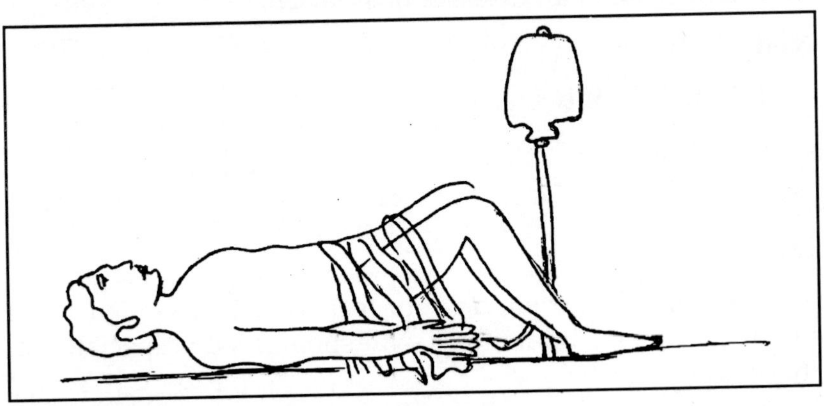

Suspend the enema pot one metre above. Apply a little oil or vaseline to the nozzle of the rectal tube. Before insertion, check the rectal tube to ensure free flow of water. Insert the tube into the rectum. The flow of water can be adjusted with the knob attached to the tube. When all the water has been introduced, remove the tube and resist the pressure for a few minutes. The bowels can be emptied after a while for better cleansing. If one does not wish to take enema in the lying position he can take it in the standing position.

Special note— Enema should be taken after going to latrine. Salt can be mixed in water instead of lemon juice. You can use plain water also. Soap should not be mixed in water.

Precautions

- Enema should be taken once in a week or in a month by a healthy person.
- It can be taken for two to four days daily in constipation.
- Take rest for half an hour after enema.
- Do not take any thing after enema for an hour.

Benefits

- Removes constipation.
- Cleans bowels.
- Beneficial in all diseases of stomach.

Neti

It is mainly of two types :

- Jala Neti
- Sutra Neti.

Jala Neti

For doing this, squat on your feet. Take tepid salted water in a medium sized pot along with spout, made especially for this purpose.

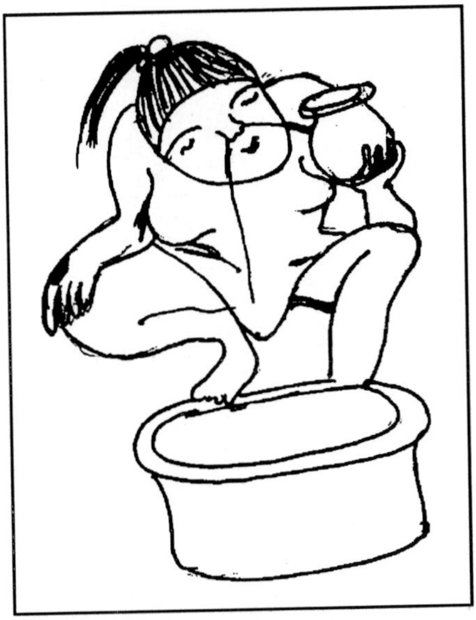

Now fill the pot with tepid salted water and hold it in your right hand to the level of your nose. Then tilt your head slightly to the left so as to have the slanting position of the left nostril. Insert the nozzle of the spout into the right nostril and allow the water to flow down slowly. The water should continue falling down from the other nostril in a continuous thin stream. Now repeat the process from the other side. Breathe through the mouth only till the kriya is complete. After Jal Neti, stand erect with your feet together. Keep the hands behind your back clasped and blow out vigorously whatever trace of water that has remained in your nostrils.

Precautions

- If sometimes one feels intolerable pain in the back of ear or above nostrils, he should practise the Kriya of Kapalbhati at once. It will cure the pain.
- Water can come out of eyes in beginning of Neti. These can be warmed. Do not fear.

Benefits

- It cures sinusitis and clears sinuses.
- It cures diseases of nose, eyes, throat and prevents the occurrence of diseases.
- It purifies mind.
- It improves memory.
- It cures coryza and removes old accumulated phlegm.

Sutra Neti or Rubber Neti

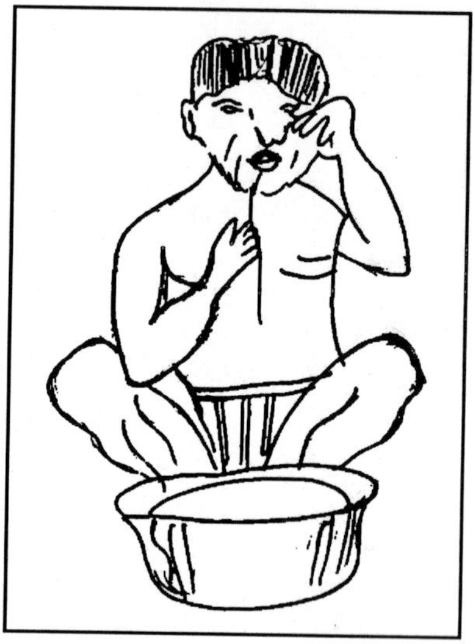

Sutra Neti is performed with a 12 inches long piece of waxed cord. It is partly twisted and it makes the nasal insertion possible.

Squat on your feet. Take tepid salted water and soak the Neti well in it. Now take the waxed and twisted end of the cord and make it to curve. Bend your head slightly forward and insert the end of the cord into the nostril through which you have been breathing at that time. Push the cord gradually through the nose, down the throat. Now open your mouth wide, put your index and middle fingers in and with their tips catch the inside end of the cord and draw it out. Hold both the ends in your hand separately and pull the cord very gently up and down three to four times. Then take it out, wash it and then repeat the cycle with the other nostril.

After completion of the kriya, wash the cord with soap well and leave it to dry in some clean and safe place so that the flies, etc. do not pollute it.

Special note

1. When the cord reaches throat through nostrils, it becomes greasy by mucus. Therefore, both the ends of the cord should be caught firmly.
2. Sutra Neti or Rubber Neti should be practised after learning Jal Neti. After this one can practise Neti with milk, oil or ghee.
3. It is more beneficial to perform this Sutra Neti by cotton cord but it should be wrapped.

Precautions

- One can sneeze in practising Sutra Neti. Water can come out of eyes. One should not fear. Practise makes one perfect.
- Nose can bleed sometimes while performing Sutra Neti. In such conditions use rubber catheter (No. 4) instead of cotton cord. Move the cord through nostrils and throat slowly and gently.

Benefits

- It cures all diseases of nose.
- It reduces polyp in nose.
- It cures sinusitis.
- It cures coryza.
- It improves eyesight.
- It improves memory.
- It purifies mind.

Nasapan

Drinking water through nostrils is called nasapan. One should clean the nostrils before drinking water through them.

Milk Neti

Milk is used in place of water. Milk should be without cream.

Benefits

Nasapan prevents cold and coryza. It improves eyesight.

Oil Neti

Warm mustard oil in a spoon. When it is lukewarm and tolerable to the skin, lie down on a bed and drip five or seven drops of oil through some dropper in both the nostrils and try to draw them in. You will feel the oil going in. You can use clean cotton instead of dropper. Coconut or almond oil can be used in place of mustard of. Pure ghee can also be used. Three or four drops of ghee or Bhadan Ragan are sufficient for the nostrils.

Oil Neti should be done before going to bed at night.

Benefits

It lubricates noses and cleanses it. It prevents from cold and coryza.

Tratak

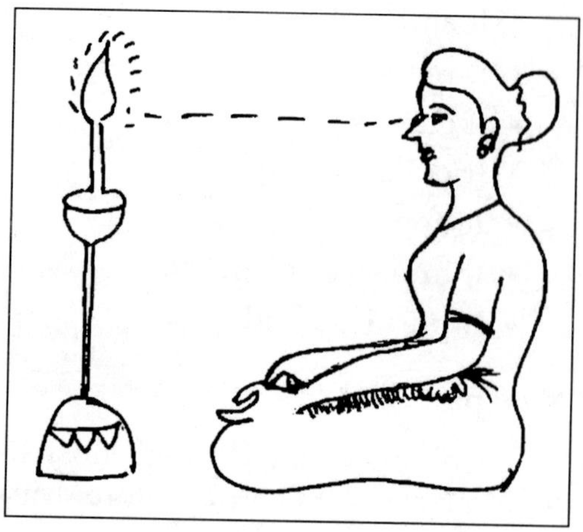

It is an amazing exercise to improve your power of concentration and eyesight.

It can be practised with a candle or with a black dot on a piece of paper fixed on the wall. Start this practice in a closed room, as there will be less objects to disturb your concentration.

Sit on floor in any comfortable pose. Keep your back and spinal cord erect. Have a few deep breaths. Make your breath steady, even and rhythmic. Keep the object of your gaze at your eye level at a distance of three to four feet. Keep the eyes meditatively wide out of your eyes. Close the eyes to let tears trickle down.

Now mentally visualizing any object open your eyes and start gazing afresh. Do not strain your nerves and get relaxed. Let not your mind wander. Try to bring your mind back to the object but without straining yourself much as that would sap your energy and you will be tired soon.

After practising with the point on the walls or on a steady flame, try to-do it concentrating on the tip of your nose on the point between the eyebrows.

Benefits

- Tratak improves eyesight and removes the diseases of eyes.
- It helps in concentrating your mind and keeps away from hurry.
- It purifies your mind.
- Once, mind is purified the digestion also becomes normal.

Nauli Kriya

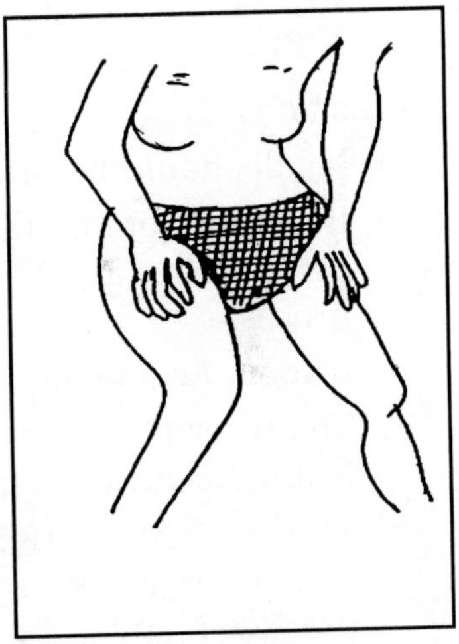

It is the best exercise for preserving and promoting the health of abdominal viscera.

- Nauli is equal to Uddiyana Bandh.
- Nauli should be practised daily in the morning on empty stomach and evacuated bowels.
- Stand with legs one foot apart. Bend the legs a little and stoop forward. Rest the palms on thighs just above your knees, with fingers spread. Press the thighs well with your palms and the chest with your chin at the notch between the collar bones.
- Inhale deeply and exhale vigorously so as to force out all the air from the lungs.
- Suspend the breath and pull the abdominal region back towards the spine so that a hollow is formed.

- Push the abdominal recti forward so that a vertical ridge down the centre is formed. Remain in this position for a few seconds and then relax the gap and inhale smoothly.
- Breathe deeply three to four times and then repeat the cycle. Repeat it five to seven times.

Special note

- Nauli kriya is not easy. Obese persons feel difficulty in its practise. It is essential to practice Uddiyana Bandh and Agnisar to perform Nauli.
- Nauli kriya should be performed on empty stomach after cleaning bowels and before taking food.
- One should wear only undergarments while practising Nauli.

Precautions

- Nauli should be practised on empty stomach.
- It should not be practised unless there is some expert to demonstrate and then to guide and supervise the whole process.
- It should not be practised before the age of 12 or 13 years.
- The ulcer patient and the weak person should perform Nauli on the advice of Yoga therapist.
- The patients suffering from swelling of intestines, dysentery, hernia and high blood pressure should not practice Nauli.

Benefits

The benefits of Nauli are many. It strengthens the abdominal muscles and liver. Women who suffer from a menstrual problem get immediate relief. It increases gastric fire and helps eliminating the toxic elements from the digestive system. It also helps in ovarian insufficiency. Nauli quickly cures constipation, dyspepsia, flatulence etc.

Kapalbhati

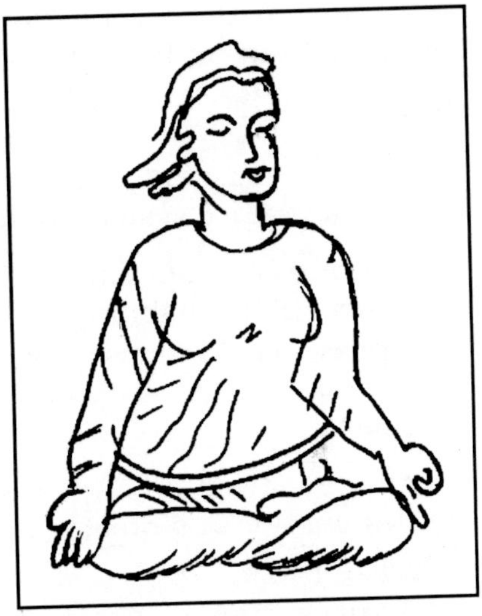

Kapal means skull. Bhati means shine or lustre. Thus, this term means "skull shining". Kapalbhati is a Pranayama also besides one of the six cleaning exercises. Actually this kriya or cleansing process is a milder form of Bhastrika , another vigorously breathing exercise.

Sit on a blanket in Padmasana, Sidhasana or Sukhasana. Keep back, spinal cord and neck erect. Keep both the hands on knees. Shut your eyes. Sit peacefully. Exhale vigorously. Do not inhale. At start begin slowly after four to five exhales exhale vigorously and quickly. Be careful in exhaling; you will inhale between exhales.

One should not pause during the practice of Kapabhati. Hold the breath after exhaling (Kumbhak). During Kumbhak practice Jallandhar Bandh, Uddiyana Bandh, Mool Bandh and Mahabandh. Hold this position for a while. Release all Bandhs and inhale slowly. This completes one round of Kapalbhati. Start with two rounds. You can practice unto five rounds gradually. Start with ten or twelve exhales. Gradually you can increase their number 50 to 120.

Special Note

1. The stomach should go inside at once after exhaling.
2. The difference between Kapabhati and Bhasrika Pranayam is that both inhale and exhale are done vigorously. One should learn it from an expert in Yogic Kriya.

Precautions

Persons with high blood pressure problems or pus in the ear should refrain from doing this exercise.

Benefits

This is very good invigorating exercise which cleanses the entire respiratory system by forcefully rushing exhalation.

It removes concentration and mental retention. The movement of the diaphragm stimulates the stomach, heart liver and spleen. This exercise is very good for eyes.

Agnisar

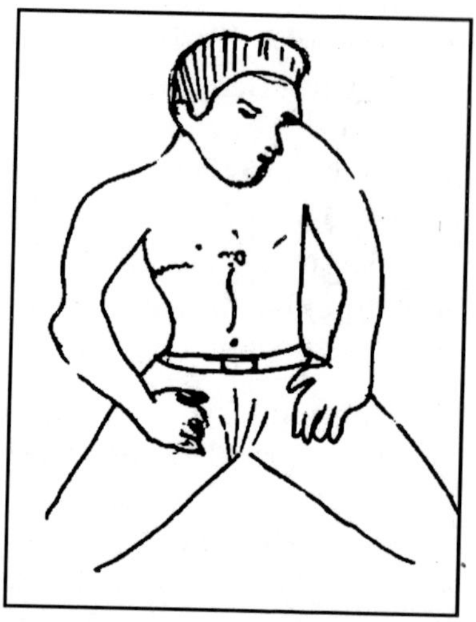

The practice of Agnisar kindles energy in stomach and body perspires.

Sit on a blanket or dari in Vajrasana. Keep a little distance between the knees. Put firmly both the hands on the knees. Inhale vigorously and while exhaling shrink your stomach as much as you can. Now suspend your breath. It is called Bahya Kumbhak.

Holding the position of Bahya Kumbhak, *i.e.* keeping the breath suspended and pulling the entire abdominal region back towards your spine. Now blow your stomach out and shrink in . In one Kumbhak you can blow and shrink your stomach 8-20 times .

This kriya is called Agnisar. One can practice this kriya in a standing posture.

Benefits

- Cures obesity.
- Cures disorders of abdominal region.
- It improves lack of appetite.

Bandh

Bandh means binding. Bandhs literally means a lock, bondage or joining together to objects or stages. A Bandh is a special posture invented to conserve and make greater use of vast resources of energy generated by yogic exercises and Pranayama. These Bandhs are means of reorientation and control of the vital energy of your body and mind. These are of three main types.

Jalandhar Bandh

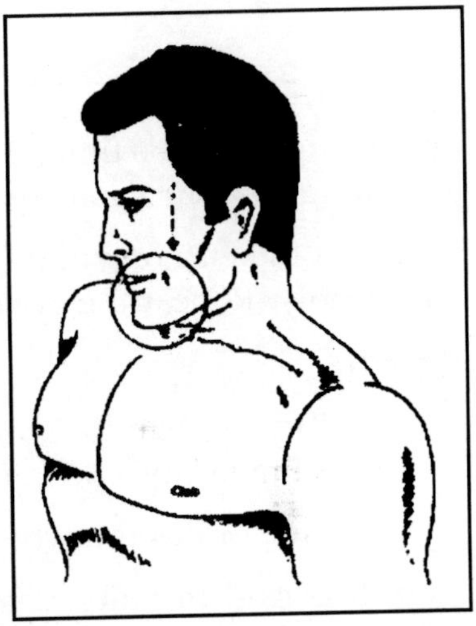

In this Bandh the throat is constantly blocked, as it were, by making the chin rest on the chest in the notch between the collar bones in certain asanas or posture like Sarvangasana exhalation and fresh, when the breath is suspended. Once in a day early in the morning it should be practised, first standing, then in advanced stage in the sitting position.

Stand erect with your feet one foot apart. Bend the knees a little and then slightly bend forward. Rest your palms with fingers spread on your thigh above the knees. Take a few deep breaths and then exhale forcefully. This is automatically practised. In these postures the chin is firmly pressed against the chest. This chin lock regulates the flow of blood to the heart, head, brain and neck. Jalandhar Bandh is also practised in combination with Mula Bandh.

Uddiyana Bandh

It is a very powerful Bandh and a basic for regulating the flow of prana and awakening of Kundalini. Uddiyana involves the lifting of the diaphragm high up the chest and pulling up

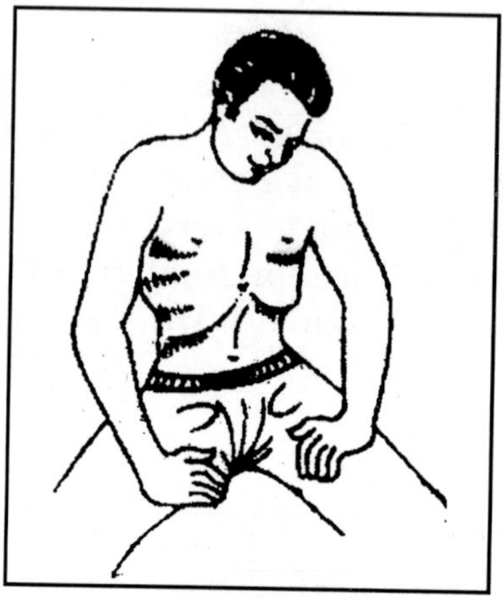

the abdominal organs towards the spine. It means to fly up . This Bandh makes the great bird of Prana fly towards the highest chakra Brahmarandhara or Sahasara. Inhale upto fill and exhale so as to empty your lungs completely.

Keep the breath suspended and pull the entire abdominal region back towards your spine. Then draw it up toward thorax. Keep the pressure of your palms on the thighs all this time. Remain in the pose for 20-30 seconds according to your capacity.

Relax the grip on your abdominal region and inhale slowly and deeply. Repeat the cycle three to five times.

Benefits

- Uddiyana Bandh is of great spiritual value as it forces the Prana upto Sushumna nadi.
- It invigorates the whole abdominal region.
- It is said to rejuvenate, if it is properly and constantly practised.
- The uplifting of diaphragm massages the heart muscles.

Mula Bandh

Mula literally means the root, source, foundation or the basis. In it the portion between anus and scrotum is contracted and raised. This prevents Apana escaping from the lower body and draws it up to unite with Prana.

Sit in Padmasana or Sidhasan. Stretch your hands and fingers as if in Gyan mudra. Now inhale deeply and retain your breath. Press the chin against the chest in the chin lock. Now contract the region of lower abdomen between the anus and the navel towards your spine and pull it upwards towards the diaphragm. Remain in the posture for a few seconds. Now release the grip on abdominal muscles and remove the chin lock. Exhale slowly and evenly. Repeat the cycle three to five times.

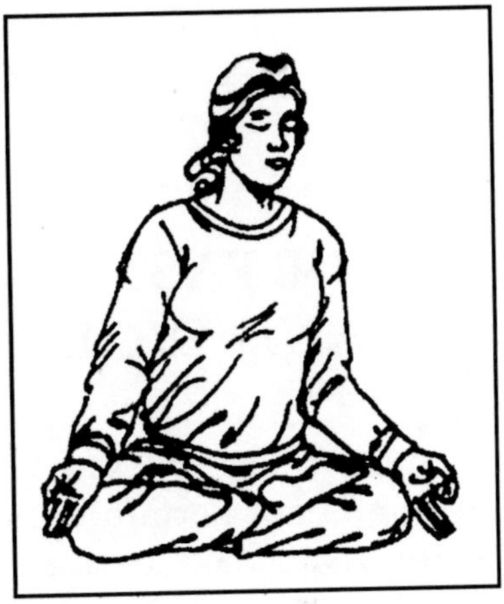

Benefits

- It cures piles.
- It cures the disorders of intestines.
- It prevents Apana vayu (foul wind) escaping from the lower body unite with the Prana vayu (the vital wind).
- It increases sexual retention power which when sublimated a man 'Urdhuvaretus' or a person of great moral and spiritual power.
- It also helps in awakening the dormant Kundalini.

The Mula Bandh should be practised when one becomes perfect in doing certain difficult asanas like Sirshansa, Sarvasana etc.

Maha Bandh

Sit in Padmasana on a blanket. Shut your eyes. Now practise Jalandhar, Uddiyaana and Mula Bandh together.

Benefits

- You get the benefits of all the three Bandhs at once by Maha Bandh.
- It cures menstrual and ovarian problems.
- It helps in strengthening sex organs of males.

■

11

JUICE FAST FOR DETOXIFICATION AND DIGESTIVE DISORDERS

Juice fasting is a safe and easy way to detoxify the body. Fasting is not harmful. Fasts have been recorded in ancient history, and have been a part of virtually all religions. for example, in the orthodox Christian church, fasts have been practised for centuries and are still a way of church life today. Fasts play an important role in Indian life too.

We do not recommend water fasts because they are too hard on the body. Such fasts release too many stored-up toxinswithout supplying the nutrients, especially the antioxidants (beta-carotene, vitamins C and E, and the mineral selenium) supplied in abundance in the juices, bind with harmful toxins and carry them out of the body.

Some words of caution are in order regarding juice fasting. Children under seventeen should not follow a strict juice fast. But fruit and vegetable juices are a great supplement to a healthful diet for your child or adolescent. Diabetics should seek a doctor's approval before trying a juice fast. Hypoglycemics may benefit from using protein powder as a supplement during the fast. Whenever your are sick, your body is sending you a signal that it needs rest—both from strenuous work and from foods that are hard to digest along with plenty of immune supporting nutrients. Juices offer great quantities of nutrients that support your immune system, and the juice fast is a powerful healing tool. But don't wait until you are sick to try fasting! We suggest a juice fast several times a year. You can fast from one to five days any time you like. Some people do a two or three-days cleansing fast every month. If you fast for longer than five days. We suggest you seek qualified supervision.

Drinks that are especially cleansing on the juice fast include beets (not more than three ounces should be consumed the first day, but this amount can be increased gradually upto six ounces), cabbage, wheat grass, sprouts, lemon, carrot, celery, and apple. In addition, you can add herbal teas such as dandelion root and nettle. These two herbs help cleanse the liver and kidneys. (Put ½ teaspoon of each herb in a pint of water, strain, and drink warm. Add lemon for flavour). Vegetable broths can be drunk as well. Gently simmer fresh vegetables with onions and garlic, strain out the vegetables. and add a dash of seasoning to make a nutritious broth you can drink as desired. Also, if you find that you need something to munch on, don't hesitate to modify the fast by adding fresh raw vegetables.

Bulking agents such as psyllium seeds husks are used commonly as mucilaginous bulk laxatives. One or two teaspoons can be added to a glass of juice once or twice a day. This can be a very helpful aid to elimination during the cleansing fast.

Breaking the fast properly is as important as the fast itself. If the fast is broken incorrectly, more bad than good can result. Actually, your diet the day before the fast should consist of raw fruits and vegetables with vegetable broths, homemade vegetable soups, or steamed vegetables. No animal products should be consumed until the second day after the fast, when fish as well as whole grains maybe added.

The suggested menu, below, is a guideline for the juice fast, which can be followed for one to five consecutive days. This schedule can be modified whenever necessary to meet your individual needs.

Recipes for Juice Fast

The following recipes offer possibilities for each "juice meal" of the day. You can choose from one of these recipes or you can make up your own. Feel free to dilute any or all of these juice receipes with water. In fact, many health professionals recommend diluting all fruit juices with an equal amount of water. Finally, we recommend that you have one beet juice and one cabbage juice drink per day because of their effectiveness in cleansing the body.

BREAKFAST

Energy Shake

A Handful of parsley
4-6 carrots, greens removed
Parsley sprig for garnish.

Bunch up parsley and push through chopper with carrots. Garnish with sprig of parsley.

Ginger Hopper

¼ inch slice ginger root, 4-5 carrots, greens removed, ½ apple, seeded.

Push ginger through chopper with carrots and apple.

Pink Morning Tonic

1 pink grapefruit, peeled
(leave white pithy part)
1 red apple, seeded

Push grarefruit through chopper with apple.

Peach Nectar

2 firm peaches, pitted
½ lime
1 ripe banana
1 tablespoon brewer's yeast.

Juice peaches and lime. Place juice, banana, and yeast in blender, and blend until smooth.

Morning Energizer

Handful parsley
5 carrots, greens removes
½ apple, seeded.

Bunch up parsley and push through chopper with carrots and apple.

MID-MORNING SNACKS

Green Surprise

1 large kale leaf
2-3 green apples, seeded
Lime twist for garnish.

Bunch up kale leaf and push through hopper with apples. Garnish with lime twist.

Cherie's Cleanising Cocktail

¼ inch slice ginger root
1 beet
½ apple, seeded
4 carrots, greens removed

Push ginger, beet, and apple through chopper with carrots.

Blood Regenerator

Handful spinach
4 lettuce leaves
4 sprigs parsley
6 carrots, greens removed
¼ turnip.

Bunch up spinach, lettuce, and parsley, and push through chopper with carrots and turnip.

Lung Tonic

Small handful parsley
4 sprigs watercress
¼ potato, peeled
6 carrots, greens removed.

Bunch up parsley and watercress, and push through chopper with potato and carrots.

LUNCH

Zippy Spring Tonic

Handful dandelion greens (unsprayed)
3 pineapple rings, without skin
3 radishes.

Bunch up dandelion greens and push through chopper with pineapple and radishes.

Potassium Broth

Handful plarsley
Handful spinach
4-5 carrots, greens removed
2 stalks celery

Bunch up parsley and spinach leaves, and push through chopper with carrots and celery.

Year-Round Cleansing Cocktail

2 parsley sprigs
Small handful wheat grass
4-6 carrots, greens removed
2 stalks celery
1 apple, seeded
½ beet

Bunch up parsley and wheat grass, and push through chopper with carrots, celery, apple and beet.

Harvest Soup

2-3 garlic cloves
1 kale leaf
1 large tomato
2 stalks celery
1 collard leaf, chopped
1 tablespoon croutons

Roll garlic in kale leaf and push through chopper with tomato and celery. Place juice in saucepan, add chopped collards, and gently heat. Garnish with croutons.

MID-AFTERNOON SNACKS

Spicy Tonic

¼ pineapple, with skin
½ apple, seeded
½ inch sliced ginger root.

Push pineapple through chopper with apple and ginger.

Digestive Special

Handful spinach
4-5 carrots, greens removed.

Bunch up spinach and push through chopper with carrots.

Liver Mover

1 small beet
2-3 apples, seeded.

Push beet and apples through chopper.

HAPPY HOUR

Watermelon Juice

2- inch slice watermelon, with rind
Orange slice for garnish.

Juice watermelon. Pour juice into glass and garnish with orange slice..

R Berry Cocktail

1 large bunch grapes
1 quart blueberries or blackberries
Sparkling water
Lemon twist for garnish

Push grapes and berries through hopper. Juice directly into small, ice-filled pitcher. Pour juice into tall glass and fill glass to top with sparkling water. Garnish with lemon twist.

DINNER

Cleansing Tonic

½ inch wedge green cabbage
2 green apples, seeded
6 carrots, greens removed

Push cabbage, apples, and carrots through chopper.

Alkaline Special

¼ head cabbage (red or green)
3 stalks celery

Push cabbage and celery through hopper.

Garden Salad Special

3 broccoli flowerets
1 garlic clove
4-5 carrots or 2 tomatoes
2 stalks celery
½ green pepper

Push broccoli and garlic through chopper with carrots or tomatoes.

Follow with celery and green pepper.

Harvest Soup

2-3 garlic cloves
1 kale leaf
1 large tomato
2 stalks celery
1 collard leaf, chopped
1 tsp. croutons.

Roll garlic in kale leaf, and push through chopper with tomato and celery. Place juice in saucepan, add chopped collards, and gently heat. Garnish with croutons.

JUICE SNACKS FOR ANY TIME OF DAY

Gingerberry Pops

1 quart blueberries
1 inch slice ginger root
1 medium bunch green grapes
3-oz. Paper cups.
Wooden popsicle sticks.

Push blueberries and ginger through chopper with grapes. Pour juice into cups, add sticks and freeze.

Berry Freeze

1 large bunch green grapes
1 large bunch red grapes
1 quart blueberries or blackberries

Juice fruit. Place juice in saucepan, add water and gently heat.

Fruit Tea

1 orange, peeled (leave while pithy part)
1 red apple, seeded.
1 lime wedge
1 auart water.

Juice fruit. Place juice in saucepan, add water, and gently heat.

High-Calcium Drink

3 kale leaves
Small handful parsley
4-5 carrots, greens removed.

Bunch up kale and parsley, and push through chopper with carrots.

Ginger Fizz

¼ inch slice ginger root
1 apple, seeded
Water.

Push ginger through hopper with apple. Pour juice into ice-filled glass. Fill glass to top with water.

Lemon Spritzer

1 small lemon

Push lemon through chopper. Pour juice into water ice-filled glass.

■

12

AYURVEDIC MEDICINES FOR DIFFERENT DIGESTIVE DISORDERS

The root of most of the diseases is stomach. We should avoid constipation and acidity by checking the wrong eating habits.

Stomach Pain Around Navel

- Grind 2 teaspoon carom seeds and dried ginger into a fine powder. Add a little black salt (kala namak). Take 1 teaspoon of this mixture with warm water frequently.

Acidity

- The best way to treat this trouble is to have lots of fresh radishes. For taste you may add carrots and tomatoes but not salt. The chlorine discharged by radish is very effective to clear the extra acidic contents from the blood. If you like, you must add a little of rock salt to make it more tasty. Drinking juice of radish would also be very helpful. But drinking this juice immediately after extracting it because the gas it has gets lost when kept for long.
- Chewing a piece of harad is an age old remedy.
- Drink coconut water 3-4 times a day.
- Have a plateful of watermelon (tarbooz) and/or cucumber (kheera) every hour.
- Harad juice, 1-2 teaspoon daily after meals is very effective in controlling acidity. The juice can be mixed with an equal amount of amla juice for better results. To take out amla juice, grate an amla and squeeze the pulp through a clean muslin cloth to get juice.

- Take a tiny piece of jaggery (gur) every hour. Just keep it in the mouth and slowly suck it till acidity subsides.
- Take dried blossom of tulsi, rind of the neem tree, black pepper and peepal in even quantity and grind them to powder form. Take 3 gms of this powder every morning and evening with plain water. All the acidic effect of the body shall pass out with urine and sweat, but remember, never to take milk over tulsi leaves which might afflict your skin.

Dyspepsia and Indigestion

- Sometimes continued irregular food intake and heavily spiced food create a positive dislike for food. Radish has not only the quality of clearing the bowels but it is a very good appetiser also. Have its pieces as much as you want, after properly adding rock salt and lemon. At this state, drinking, radish juice would not be as effective as to have raw radish, skip your meal and have only salads soon you'd long for food.
- Boil 5-6 sticks of powdered cinnamon in a glass of water. Add a pinch of pepper powder and little honey. A tablespoon of the above concoction take 1/2 hour after meals relieves indigestion and flatulence (gas).
- Mix 1/4 teaspoon pepper powder, 1/4 teaspoon of cumin (jeera) powder to a glass of buttermilk. Have this 1-2 times a day.
- A golden rule to avoid indigestion; get up from the dining table when you can still eat some more or are a little hungry. Chew food well.
- Add 1 teaspoon fresh grated ginger (adrak) to 1 cup water. Cover and simmer on low heat for 5 minutes. Strain and drink 1-2 times a day.
- Soak one teaspoon of celery seeds in a glass of butter milk for 5-6 hours. Grind in the same buttermilk and drink it 1-2 times a day.

(i) Mix about 6 gms. of castor oil with 20 gms of milk to clean the bowels.

(ii) Take roasted borax 3 gms. Bishop's seeds 3 gms, Kala Namak 3 gms, grind them to the powdered and pass through from the sieve or through a thick cloth. Administer 2 gms. of the powder everyday with lukewarm water.

- Mix 1 teaspoon mint juice, 1 teaspoon lemon juice, juice of 1/4 piece ginger and a pinch of black salt (kala namak) and drink it.
- Mix a little asafoetida (hing) with water to make a paste. Apply on and around the navel.
- Drink 1-2 teaspoons brandy with a little warm water. Gives immediate relief from gas.
- Mix carom seeds (ajwain) with lemon juice and dry in the sun. Bottle it and have a teaspoon whenever you feel that something is wrong with your stomach (very good for stomach digestion, gas, indigestion etc.)
- And then there is the age old method of using a hot water bottle and lying down on your somach to get relief.
- Swallow with warm water, 1 teaspoon carom seeds (ajwain) and pinch of salt.
- 1 teaspoon pure ghee mixed with a pinch of asafoetida (hing), swallow with warm water.

Indigestion

- Take the seeds of tulsi and peepal in equal quantity and grind them to fine powder form. Now add 3 gms. of this powder with a spoonful of honey and lick it twice a day to clear indigestion.
- Drinking the tea of tulsi leaves also brings quick relief. The filthy substance will get out of the body with sweat and urine. Alternatively add 1 gm. of rock salt in 10 gms. of tulsi leaves' paste and swallow it down with water.

Stomach Burn

- Take 1 teaspoon fenugreek seeds (methi daana), powder along with milk or buttermilk twice daily for a few days.

Stomach Heaviness

- Mix ¼ teaspoon powdered cumin (jeera) seeds and black peeper in a glass of buttermilk (chhach). Drink two or three times a day for 2-3 days.

Abdominal Pain

- Add ½ teaspoon camphor (kapoor) and 1 tablespoon sandalwood paste to 1 tablespoon warm mustard oil. Massage gently over the lower abdomen.

Colic in Babies

- Boil a teaspoon of fennel seeds (saunf) in a cup of water. Boil for 2-3 minutes and keep it to cool for 15-20 minutes. Strain it. Add 1-2 teaspoon to every feed of milk of the baby. It helps cure colic.

Constipation

It can be caused by many reasons, the prime one being wrong eating habits of the person and wrong choice of food also. The following treatments are quite effective:

- Soak the pith of Amaltas 50 gms. overnight and strain the water in the morning to drink it adding 20 gms. of sugar.
- Have a glass of water with a spoonful of honey added to it every night before you go to sleep.
- Take cumin seeds 20 gms; dry ginger 20 gms; white cumin seeds 20 gms; ammounium chloride 5 gms; small cardamom 5 gms; bishop's seed (ajwain) 20 gms; pippli 10 gms; black pepper 10 gms., cloves 5 gms; asafoetida 5 gms; old jaggery 50gms; musk camphor 2 gms. Grind

and sieve all the ingredients after mixing together and keep the powder in a glass vessel. Then grind the powder again with the juice of ginger. Then grind it again with the juice of lemon. Add more lemon juice if dries up. Grind the mixture well for 15 days and then dry it in shade. Dry it as much as to facilitate your making small balls out of the grind paste. For any stomach disorder have two of these tablets daily with water after meals to get rid of any stomach ailment.

- Take a glass of warm water with 1 teaspoon honey and juice of ½ a lemon, as first thing in the morning.
- Soak 6-8 dates (khajoor) in a cup of water at night . Churn in the mixer in the morning and drink in the morning.
- Consume approx. 250-300 gms. fresh grapes (angoor) everyday. When grapes are not in season, soak 12-15 raisins (kishmish) in water and have them. Raisins should be soaked for 24-48 hours and eaten early in the morning. The water in which they are soaked should also be drunk.
- Simply eat a few liquorice (mulathi) sticks. One of its many properties is that it is a natural laxative.

Constipation in Small Children

- Whole wheat flour should be used and processed foods (maida, cheese, confectionery) should be avoided.
- Taking 2-3 teaspoons of isabgol in milk or warm water at bed time is very beneficial.
- Mix ½ teaspoon honey to ½-1 cup warm water and have it 2-3 times a day.
- Soak 6-8 raisins in hot water (depending on the age). When cool, crush well and strain. When given routinely even to infants, it helps to regulate bowel movement (however care should be taken so as not to give too much otherwise the child might get loose motions).

- Consumption of 6-8 apricots(khumani) a day or 2-3 cucumbers (kheera) a day or 1-2 bananas a day is also very useful.
- Bulk forming vegetables like carrots, radish, spinach, cabbage or roughage creating things should be consumed. Instead of juice always opt for eating the fruit.
- The best way to treat this common problem is to have lots of fresh radish with black salt or rock-salt and lemon juice sprinkled on them. Radish is an ideal purgative. If one takes half a cup of fresh radish juice as the first thing in the morning it is still better. Don't eat anything till you have constipation. If possible have very light diet and eat radish as salad. If you have a little piece of jaggery over the radish diet, even the foul smell shall be considerably subsided.

Loose Motions

When the system fails to digest the rich food, the body rejects it as it is in the form of the loose motion. Try the following treatments:

- Give about 5 gms. of Isabgol with cold water in which about 1 teaspoonful sugar has been added.
- Peel an apple and shred it. Keep the shredded pieces in a plate for approximately 20 minutes until they turn brown in colour and then eat them.
- Slice the tender unripe bel fruit. Sundry them. Powder the slices. Take 1 teaspoon along with warm water twice a day.
- Take every night. 3 cloves of garlic (lahasun), chopped and boiled in milk.
- Make a paste of 1 green chilli along with 2 tablespoon lime juice and 1/2 teaspoon camphor (kapoor). Take 1/4 teaspoon of this paste.
- 2 or 3 teaspoons coriander seeds (sabot dhania) soaked overnight in water and take next morning with 1 cup buttermilk (chhach).

- Boil 1/4 teaspoon powdered cardamom (chhoti ilaichi) seeds in thin tea water and drink.
- Mix juice of 15-20 tender curry leaves (curry patta) with 1 teaspoon honey and drink.
- Apply ginger (adrak) juice around the navel.
- Combine 1 teaspoon each powdered ginger (adrak) powdered cumin (jeera) and powdered cinnamon (dalchini) with honey and make into a thick paste. Take 1 teaspoon thrice daily.
- Boil 1 teaspoon cumin seeds (jeera) in a glass of water. Add to this 1 teaspoon fresh juice of coriander leave (dhania) and a pinch of salt. Drink twice daily after meals for 2-3 days.
- Mash 1 ripe banana along with a pinch of salt and 1teaspoon tamarind pulp (imli ka guda). Take twice a day.
- Drinking unsweetened black tea is very effective for stopping diarrhoea.

For Children

- Ripe and sweet apples crushed to a pulp (can be steamed) can be given as 1-4 tablespoon several times a day.
- Mashed ripe banana with a little salt, should be taken 2-3 times a day.
- A teaspoon of date (khajoor) paste mixed with a little honey, given three times a day is very effective for regulating the bowels.
- 5-10 gms of amla seed powder mixed with buttermilk (chhach) should be taken for 1-2 days.
- Crush 8-10 curry leaves (curry patta). Mix with a cup of thin buttermilk (chhach) and have 2-3 times a day.
- Mix juice of 1 large pomegranate (anar) and 1 glass of sugarcane juice (ganne ka ras). Have 4 times a day.

- A fast with only buttermilk, curd, curd and rice or bananas proves very effective.
- Avoid raw vegetables and fruits such as orange, sweet lime, papaya, pineapple and spices.
- Drink plenty of water to which a teaspoon of sugar and a pinch of salt has been added to guard against dehydration.
- A strong cup of unsweetened black tea is very effective.

Stools With Blood

- 1 tablespoon juice of the flower of pomegranate (anar) with sugar candy (mishri), taken twice daily.

Dehydration

- Soak half a nutmeg (jaiphal) in 2 cups water for over 2-3 hours. Take 1 teaspoon of this infusion and mix in 1 cup fresh coconut water, drink thrice a day.

Cholera

This epidemic occurs in hot and humid season. It is invariably accompanied by frequent loose motions and loss of weight. If not treated in due time, this disease could be fatal. The remedies to check this disease are the following.

- Administer opium 5gms. in 10 gms. of edible lime to stop the loose motion.
- Grind the lemon seeds and mix it in rose water. Administer it orally for quick relief.
- Pull out the root of the plant swallow work(Aak in Hindi), clean the dirt from it and unpeel its rind. Add the black pepper with equal amount of this rind and form a paste of them. Then roll out small tablets. Administer each tablet with water at the interval of two hours.
- Take fresh mint leaves and grind them with small cardamoms. Boil both of them in water and thicken the

fluid by heat. When the fluid is thick and homogeneous, let the patient sip it as and when he desires it. Give lot of water to the patient to drink. Keep his clothes and beds clean. The affected patient must stay aloof.

Flatulence and Belching

- Soak 3 tablespoons carom (ajwain) seeds in an adequate quantity of lime juice and dry in the shade. When fully dried, powder with a little black salt. Take 1 teaspoon of this mixture twice daily for a few days with a little warm water. (This treatment is more effective when fats and spices are avoided in the diet.)
- Grind 2 teaspoons each carom seeds and dried ginger into a fine powder. Add a little black salt. Take 1 teaspoon of this mixture with 1 cup warm water frequently.
- Powder together dry ginger with black pepper, equal amounts, say 1 teaspoon each and 3-4 cardamom (chooti illaichi) seeds. Have 1/2 teaspoon of this mixed with water to relieve gas.
- Apply a paste of asafoetida (hing) mixed with water on the stomach.
- Make a coarse powder (churan) of equal amounts of cumin seeds (jeera), carom seeds (ajwain), black pepper corns (saboot kali mirch) and fenugreek seeds (methi daana). Have 1/2 teaspoon with water.
- To prevent gas from forming, chew a piece of fresh ginger after meals regularly.
- Add a teaspoon of caraway seeds to 1½-2 litres of water and boil it on low flame for 15 minutes. Strain and drink 1 cup of this tea, hot or warm 3 times a day after meals.
- A drop of dill oil (soye ka tel) mixed with a teaspoon of honey, licked immediately after meals is very effective in controlling gas.

- Wash black harad well with water and wipe with a clean dry cloth, store in a air tight bottle. Suck one piece after meals. Keep in the mouth till it dissolves completely. This is effective in controlling gas and constipation
- Mix ¼ teaspoon dry ginger powder (sonth) with a pinch of asafoetida (hing) and a pinch of black salt (rock salt) (kala namak) in a little warm water and drink it.
- Mix 1-2 teaspoons brandy with warm water and drink for immediate relief from gas and stomach ache due to gas.
- Some people are allergic or have intolerance for milk, milk products and wheat, wheat products, but go through life without ever realizing this and keep suffering from acute gas trouble. Lactose intolerance (from milk) is being recognized in the west as also gluten intolerance (from wheat). Hence giving up these two things may greatly benefit you. Instead of wheat you can have rice or chapatis of maize, jawar or bajara.
- Take Bishop's seeds, 10 gms., dry ginger 6 gms., kala namak 3 gms., grind them well to powder form and administer thrice daily with water. Take 3 gms. of powder each time.
- Munch your food properly and eat slowly, without letting air enter your system when you gulp your food.'
- Take a spoonful of ginger juice, add salt and take it after your meals.
- Take dry ginger, Bishop's seeds, and about 2 spoonfuls of lemon juice. Mix them well and take the combination whenever you have a feeling of overfulness or any gastric trouble.
- Asaoetida should be an essential condiment of your food if you have this trouble. If you feel pain in your stomach, rub asafoetida added to water over and around your navel.

Hiccups

- Grind 4 cardamom (chhoti illaichi) well. Boil it in 2½ cups or ½ litre water. When about 1 cup water remains, remove from fire and sieve it through a muslin cloth. Let it cool. When warm, drink a glassful. It works like magic.
- Suck 2-3 small pieces of fresh ginger (adrak). This helps in hiccups which keep occurring again and again.
- Drink ½ glass water, slowly.
- Keep a teaspoon of sugar in your mouth and suck slowly.
- Swallow ½ teaspoon mustard seeds mixed with ½ teaspoon pure ghee.
- Take five gms. of turmeric and five gms. of Urad pulse. Grind them to fine powder, put them in a live chilum and take a long puff. The hiccups trouble will be instantly cured.

Nausea and Vomiting

- Mix ½ teaspoon of fresh ginger (adrak) juice with 1 teaspoon each of fresh lime, mint (pudina) juice and 1 tablespoon of honey and drink.
- Slice a ripe banana, sprinkle some powdered sugar and freshly grind cardamoms (chhoti illaichi) on top. Eat 1-2 times a day.
- Eat ½ teaspoon grind cumin seeds (jeera).
- Ginger (adrak) tea or sucking sliced ginger (adrak) work by interrupting nausea signals sent from the stomach to the brain. If you are a herbal tea drinker simply sprinkle powdered cinnamon on the tea and drink. To make ginger tea, simmer a few slices of ginger in hot tea water .

Vomiting due to Indigestion

- Frequent intake of lime juice is a good remedy.
- Licking the powder of fried cloves (laung) mixed with honey controls vomiting.

- Sucking a piece of ice also controls vomiting.
- Mix 2-3 teaspoon of curry leaves (curry patta) juice with a teaspoon of lime juice (can add little sugar if needed) . Drinking this will control morning sickness, nausea and vomiting.
- Crush 2-3 cloves of garlic (lahasun) and boiled with 3/4 cup of water or milk. Boil till half the amount remains and then drink. It takes care of all digestive disorders.

Worms in Stomach and Intestines

- If you have only carrot or preparation made of carrot for a few days, the worms shall vanish. The best course is to have enough of jalebi and milk combination followed by carrot pickle soaked in mustard seeds water. This treatment will centralige the wormround jalebi - milk combination and the mustard water soaked carrot would kill them and expel them out of the system.
- The smell of radish is enough to drive away even the poisonous insects let alone these worms. Just have radish juice mixed with rock salt and lemon juice twice a day, preferably after every meal. In less than three days you would find your intestines are clear of these worms. In fact, having a little of this juice after every meal is an ideal way to prevent the occurrence of these worms.
- Fry fenugreek seeds in a little ghee and grind to a powder. Store in an airtight bottle. Add some powder to drinking water and drink 2-3times daily for 2-3 days.
- Take 1 tablespoon juice extracted from bitter gourd (karela) leaves. Mix into a glassful of buttermilk and take every morning.
- Steep some cloves (laung) in ½ cup water for 6 to 8 hours and use it for enema.
- Fry 1 teaspoon dried neem flowers in 1 teaspoon ghee and mix with 1 cup boiled rice and eat twice or thrice a day.

- Slice and dry the kernel of mango. Mix 1 tablespoon fenugreek seeds (methi daana) and powder it. Take 1 teaspoon in buttermilk.
- Eat papayas frequently.
- Take 5-10 seeds of bitter gourd (karela) and crush them. Fry them in a little ghee. Take twice daily.
- Soak mustard seeds overnight or for two days and when the water turns sour give it to the patient after meals.
- Ask the patient to eat a ripe and roasted-on fire tomato as the first thing in the morning for three to four days.
- Take 25 gms. of the rind of the roots of pomegranate plant and three times boil it. When water remains half of the original quantity, strain the water and divide into three dosages. Have first dose in the morning as the first thing and the other doses after two hourly interval. Have about 10 gms. of castor oil after the laste dose. Your worms in the stomach will clear out.
- Have sour whey after your food at least twice daily for quick relief.

Haemorrhoids (piles)

Piles or haemorrhoids, is a varicose and often inflamed condition of the veins about the lower end of the bowel. The piles are either external or internal or mixed. In external piles there is not much bleeding but a lot of pain, whereas the internal piles consist in discharge of several ounces of dark blood through anus. Try the following treatments:

- Radish is an ideal antidote for this disorder. Take a cupful of radish juice and add about 5gms. of pure ghee. Mix them well with a spoon and drink this potion in the evening and in the morning.
- Take a long radish and divide in four equal parts lengthwise. Apply a little of salt and keep it in the open for the entire night so that fresh dew may fall over it.

Have it as the first thing in the morning. After passing stool, wash the anus with radish water.

- If piles are bleeding type, have masoor dal in your lunch, followed by sour but fresh whey.
- Take the kernal of Bakain seeds about 20 gms., add 6 gms of black pepper and knead them together to form tiny tablets. Have 3 gms. of the tables in the morning and 3gms. in the evening after mixing khand sugar into it.

These troubles include many ailments including enlargement of liver, bitter belches, wind trouble and the like. The main cause could be congenital, due to wrong habits or as a symptom to some other functional disturbance in the body. Try the following treatments:

- Eat radish as much as you can with your meals or afterwards. Sugarcane juice should be an essential part of your diet.
- Take two gms. of the pith of Amaltas, hari makoya, grind them to paste form and apply it over your liver region.
- Always piss while standing after your principal meals whether you feel the urge or not. Try to sleep on your leftside after your principle meals. Just take five grams of turmeric powder mixed in a glassful of separated whey every morning and evening to reactivate the sluggish liver and repair the damage.
- Take 5 tulsi leaves, 2 gms., roasted powder of cumin seeds and 2 gms. of black salt. Grind them together to make it in a homogeneous powder form. Add to it even amount of the kernal of the wood apple. Mix the combination in about 100 gms. of curd to reactivate the sluggish liver. For early relief from any sort of stomach disorder, drink a spoonful of the combination of the juices of tulsi and ginger.

Fistula

- Have three or four tulsi leaves every morning with water or put them in your water are likely to drink at least half an hour before you actually imbibe it. Alternatively take the root of tulsi plant and the fruit of neem tree (Nimboli) and grind them together. Take 2 gms. of this combination every morning with whey for quick relief.

Jaundice

- Twenty grams of leaves of heena should be steeped in water overnight. The mixture should be strained in the morning and drunk for a few days. Juice of leaves of horse radish should be boiled and strained. Twenty grams of raw sugar should be added to the mixture and drink. The yellow pigment in the eyes can be dealt effectively by grinding seven grains of small fennel in a women's milk and introduced into the nostrils.
- A fine paste of tender papaya leaves, about ½ teaspoon paste, is taken with some water.
- Pour over a handful of lime leaves in 1 cup hot water and take the infusion.
- Make a fine powder of 1 teaspoon each crushed liquorice root, chicory seeds (kaasni) and rock salt (kala namak). Take ½ teaspoon with water twice daily.
- 1 to 2 teaspoon fresh juice of coriander (dhania) leaves is mixed in 1 cup buttermilk and taken 2-3 times.
- Mash a ripe banaba along with 1 tablespoon honey and eat twice a day for a few days.
- Frequently take lime juice.
- Take ¼ teaspoon turmeric (haldi) along with a glass of hot water 2 or 3 times daily.
- ½ teaspoon ginger juice with 1 teaspoon each fresh lime and mint juice mixed with a tablespoon of honey. Take it frequently.

- Finely grind some bel leaves. Take 1 teaspoon of this paste along with a pinch of black pepper and follow it with 1 cup of butter milk thrice a day.

Yellow Pigmentation in Eyes due to Jaundice

- Grind ¼ teaspoon black cumin seeds (kala jeera) in breast milk and introduce a pinch into the nostrils.
- The main thing to be remembered in a case of jaundice is that if the liver is not burdened (through daily flushing of the intestines) and a fat free diet is taken, the organ will recover its vitality even without medication. Sweet substances and liquids like sugarcane juice, fruit juices and dry grapes should form the mainstay of a patient's diet. About 100 gms. of dried Tamarind (Imali) pith should be soaked in water overnight together with half the quantity of dried plums (allo bhukhara), mashed and the thick liquid taken by adding a little black salt to it in the morning. The patient should take as much whey as he can during the day.
- Add 10 gms. tulsi leaves juice in about 50 gms. of radish juice. Add a little of jaggery to the combination to sweeten it. Have this solution twice or thrice daily for about a month for getting total relief from this problem.
- Alternatively take 3 gms. of tulsi leaves' juice and 3 gms. of the root of punarnava. Mix them both in 50 gms. of water and drink it for about 15 days.

Flatulence

- Take about 10 gms. of tulsi juice, 10 gms. of dry ginger and 20 gms. of jaggery. Mix all of them together to form small tablets. Take this tablet thrice a day with water to set right your digestive process. But during the period you have this trouble, better keep fast or take only easily digestible food.

Piles

- Wash 2-3 dried figs (anjeer) very well and soak in a glass of cold water overnight. Have it first thing in the morning. Have them for 2-3 weeks for good results. It is effective in ordinary as well as bleeding piles.
- 3 teaspoon of the juice of the leaves of bittergourd mixed with a glassful of buttermilk taken every morning for a month is a good remedy for piles.
- The juice of radish or consuming fresh radish is very effective. The juice should be given in dose of 60-90 ml, morning and evening.
- Take ½ teaspoon each of powder of dried pomegranate flowers, poppy seeds and dried neem leaves, twice a day with milk for bleeding piles.
- Mix juice of 15-20 tender curry leaves (curry patta) with 1 teaspoon honey and drink.
- Take 1 tablespoon black cumin seeds and roast them. Mix in another tablespoon of black cumin seeds and powder them finely. Take ½ teaspoon of this powder with a glass of water everyday.

Appetite Loss (Anorexia)

- Take 2 teaspoons of amla juice and mix it with 2 teaspoon honey and 2 teaspoons lime juice. Add 1 cup water and drink on an empty stomach every morning. To take out juice from fresh amla, remove seeds from fresh amla and grind the pulp into a fine paste. Tie it in a muslin cloth and squeeze out the juice. Whenever fresh fruits are not available dried amla at night in a cup of water. Strain it the next morning. Add ⅛ teaspoon black pepper powder (kali mirch) and 2 teaspoon lime juice. Dilute it if necessary with water and drink every morning regularly on an empty stomach.

- Take ½ teaspoon black pepper powder (kali mirch) and 1 tablespoon jaggery powder (shakkar) mixed together.
- Mix half teaspoon each of carom seeds (ajwain), fennel seeds (saunf), dried ginger powder (sonth), salt and black cumin seeds (shah jeera). Swallow about 3/4 teaspoon of this mixture with water 2-3 times a day.

Dehydration

- Add 1/4 teaspoon salt, 3 teaspoon brown sugar or ordinary sugar and 2 teaspoon lime juice to 1 cup of water, mix well and drink.

■

13

HOMOEOPATHIC MEDICINES FOR DIFFERENT DIGESTIVE DISORDERS

Amoebic Dysentery

- If the person is extremely anxious and restless with diarrhea, give Arsenicum album.
- If the person has exhausting diarrhea with lots of cramping, think of Arsenicum album and Podophyllum.
- If the stool is explosive, consider Croton tiglium, Gambogia, or Podophyllum.
- If there is significant nausea and vomiting, first consider Ipecac, then Arsenicum album.
- If there is lots of rumbling and gurgling in the abdomen, give Podophyllum, Croton tiglium, or Gambogia.
- If there is profuse diarrhea and cramping with sweating and shivering, first think of Veratrum album then Arsenicum album.

Colic

- If the baby can't seem to tolerate milk, first think of Aethusa, then Magnesia phosphorica, Calcarea carbonica or Lycopodium.
- If there is a tendency toward frequent belching, and the baby seems to feel better after belching, Carbo vegetabilis is likely to be needed.
- For colic in extremely fussy, irritable babies, especially if they arch their backs and areinconsolable, consider Chamomilla.

- If a baby doubles over with the colic or brings his knees up to his chest, think of Colocynthis first then Magnesia phosphorica.
- For colic with excessive bloating and gas, particularly if the baby seems to be worse after ingesting milk, look at Magnesia phosphorica.

Constipation

For constipation that is due to dryness with no urge, in a person who seems confused, consider Alumina.

- A person who needs Bryonia has large, hard stools with dryness, and a lot of thirst for cold drinks; many symptoms are worse from motion.
- For a stubborn, chilly flabby person who sweats on his head and has stubborn constipation, try Calcarea carbonica.
- When there is dryness, and a dreamy, drowsy, dizzy state, give Nux moschata.
- When the person is an irritable businessperson, consider Nux vomica or Bryonia.
- If the person has constant urges but can't go, even with a lot of straining , try Nux vomica.
- For constipation during pregnancy and menstruation, and a feeling like a ball in the anus of that the rectum and uterus will fall out, consider Sepia.
- For bashful stool (comes out part way, then recedes) in a refined, shy person with sweaty feet, try Silica.

Diarrhoea

If stool is like jelly due to mucus, give Aloe.

- If the person is chilly, anxious, nervous and restless, Arsenicum album is your best bet.
- If diarrhoea comes immediately after eating or drinking, look at Croton tiglium and Gambogia.

- If there is a lot of rectal itching with the diarrhea, combined with urgency first thing in the morning, Sulphur is indicated.

- If the diarrhea is violent and is accompanied by profuse sweating and chills, give Veratrum album.

Gas

- If bloating is extreme or if the person is exhausted or collapsed and wants to be fanned, give Carbo vegetabilis.
- If the person is doubled over in pain and doubling over makes him feel better, give Colocynthis.
- When gas and bloating take away the appetite, and the person lacks confidence and is worse from 4:00 to 8:00 pm., give Lycopodium.
- If the person is chilly, irritable and impatient and can't seem to pass the gas without straining, give Nux vomica.
- When the person is weepy, changeable and clingy and has eaten too much fat or rich food, give Pulsatilla.

Haemorrhoids

- If the main symptom is pain like small sharp sticks in the rectum, consider Aesculus and Collinsonia.

- If swelling and bleeding are prominent, think first of Hamamelis..

- If the person is chilly, over stressed, and drinks too much alcohol, consider Nux vomica.

- In a warm blooded person with lots of the rectal itching and recal spasms, give Sulphur.

Hepatitis

- The most common medicines are Chelidonium, china and Lycopodium.

- If there is considerable right shoulder blade pain, give Chelidonium.

- If the person has a history of gonorrhea or chlamydia, he probably needs Natrum sulphuricum.
- If perspiration and the breath smell bad and there is excessive saliva, give mercurius.
- If the person has a strong craving for cold drinks, look at Phosphorus.

Indigestion

- When extreme burnig pain is the main symptom, along with a lot of anxiety and restlessness, think of Arsenicum, especially in a self centered person who wants support and has many fears.
- Lycopodium is the medicine if the person is insecure yet bossy and full of false bravado, gets lots of gas from just a little food, and is worse from 4:00 to 8:00 P.M.
- When the person is irritable, impatient and hard-driving, and suffers from too much rich food, coffee and alcohol, give Nux vomica.
- Conversely, when the person suffers from rich food, but is mild, gentle, changeable and weepy and wants to be taken care of, think of Pulsatilla.
- If the person is lazy, intellectual, egotistical and sloppy and suffers from heartburn and morning diarrhea, give Sulphur.

Nausea/Vomiting

- Ipecac is the first medicine to think of for strong nausea and vomiting.
- Use Bismuth or phosphorus when the vomiting is primarily of liquids, and they are vomited after becoming warm in the stomach.
- Nux vomica should be considered when the vomiting comes on from emotional stress, especially anger and frustration, and it is difficult for the person to vomit.

- Phosphorus can be considered for vomiting blood and for vomit that looks like coffee grounds, in a friendly, open, sympathetic person who desires cold drinks but vomits them.
- Tabacum is the best for deathly nausea and vomiting from motion, like seasickness.
- Veratrum album is useful for a combination of nausea, vomiting, and diarrhea, especially if the person is very cold but desires ice and sour foods such as lemons and pickles.

Stomach ache

- If the stomach or abdominal pain is aggravated by motion, give Bryonia.
- If doubling up relieves the pain, think of Colocynthis or Magnesia phosphorica.
- The first medicine to think of for violent cramping is Cuprum.
- If the pain is relieved by standing up straight and made worse by bending double, the best medicine is Dioscorea.
- If the person gets bloated after eating even a small amount of food, choose Lycopodium.
- If pressure relieves the pain, consider Magnesia phosphorica, but if pressure aggravates the pain, look at Lycopodium.
- For stomach or abdominal pain after too much alcohol or spicy or rich foods, first think of Nux vomica.
- A plump, gentle, moody woman who doesn't do well with rich foods is likely to need Pulsatilla.

■

14

ALLOPATHIC TREATMENT OF DIFFERENT DIGESTIVE DISORDERS

The treatment plan of different digestive disorders as per allopathic guideline is described here:

Allopathic Treatment of Constipation

- Take Isapgol, Agar-Agar or Methyl cellulose. These drugs take 12-24 hours to act, help to absorption of water so as to, increase bulk of all the three devices mentioned above.
- Isapgol husk (one tablespoon dissolved in lukewarm/hot milk) is, by far, the best and most effective medicine which can remove both recent, acute and chronic varieties of constipation.
- If Agar-Agar is preferred, its dose is 4-16 gm, and for methyl cellulose 1-6 gms, spread over a period of 24 hours.
- Consume plenty of fruit and vegetable juices or take in raw form, plenty of water and other liquids, moderate milk, ghee/ butter, whey, curd, papaya, coconut (green) water.

Stool Softeners

Cremaffin: If the above-mentioned agents fail to regulate bowels, take liquid Cremaffin to soften hard stools but it must not be taken regularly and habitually. First, continue with 2 tablespoon dose at bedtime for 3-4 days but do not continue consecutively giving a dose on each alternate day. Some patients pass loose motions which indicates softening of stools but, then the dosage should be reduced.

Liquid Paraffin: 3-5 tablespoon at night, but must not be taken regularly as it is a habit forming medicine. Use it also after operation of piles, knotty and hard stools, to remove tenesmus and pain. Its action starts after 12-24 hours, hence do not expect an instant or quick results.

Milk of Magnesia (Magnesium Hydroxide): Liquid Cremaffin contains milk of Magnesia and former is decidedly a better option. Usual dose being 2-4 gms. Its action starts after 2-6 hours. It may produce flatulence in some patients. Avoid using in chronic renal (kidney) disease.

Magnesium Sulphate: It is taken in the morning (5-10 gms.) as a single dose. But being a strong purgative, it causes total evacuation of bowels with 2-3 hours. I do not recommend it because, even if a minute quantity of it reaches blood (from intestines), it may cause depression or central nervous system, cause serious dehydration, anuria, hence it is not used these days. Instead of this, castor oil can be taken.

***Note*:** There are irritant purgatives like Bisacodyt, Phenolphthalein, Senna Glycosides etc. which deserve to be discarded due to serious side-effects.

***Caution*:** Consult your doctor while giving any purgative to an infant, child, pregnant lady, elderly, person having some serious complaints and health problems, operated cases etc.

Allopathic Treatment of Diarrhoea

Lomotil: One tablet thrice daily. It may colour the urine. Do not use for children below 10 years, pregnant ladies and elderly. Causes dryness of mouth, blurred vision, bitter taste yellow colour of urine. If taken for a longer period, it may cause addiction, respiratory depression, coma, and even death may ensue.

Furoxone: Its advantage being that it effectively controls diarrhoea and micro-organisms but do not become resistant to it. It is also of value in infections and gastro-enteritis. It is more effective than Tetracyclin, Chlorumphenicol, Sulphadiazine or

Sulphathiazole. Its usual dose is 100 mg 4 times a day. Nausea, vomiting, headache, yellow urine, skin rashes or other allergic reactions may surface but, all the same, it has minimal side effects. If nausea, vomiting or allergic reactions supervene, either taper/reduce the dose or else withdraw it.

Wotinex: Take one tablet twice daily. Do not given to children below 12, pregnant ladies and persons with liver problems. It may give bitter or coppery taste in the mouth.

Ampicillin: 250 mg 4 times daily or 500 mg twice daily. In certain patients it causes diarrhoea, hence persons with sensitive digestive system should not use it.

Neomycin: This is an antibiotic drug of choice and is specifically used for infants due to its local action. Consult some doctor for suitable and requisite dose and frequency.

Allopathic Treatment of Dysentery

☞ Tablet/Capsule of 'Nalidixic Acid (150-300 mg) + Metronidazole (200 mg). Adult dose 2-3 tab/cap 3-4 times daily, depending on intensity and severity of the case. Do not give to infants, nursing and pregnant ladies. If nausea and vomiting persist take a tablet (thrice daily) of 'Peri norm' or 'Stemitil' or' Avomine' also. Trade brand names of Nalidixic and Metronidazole being 'Bactomed', 'Enterodix-M', 'Genogyl-M, 'Microneg', Enterodix-M. Do not be scared if yellow/pale,coloured urine is passed, in addition to bitter tase in the mouth.

☞ Also try cap 'Inseptin-MF'. One tablet/cap for adults six hourly; for children over 5 years 1/2 tablet 8 hourly or as required. Urine may be passed yellow or pale, and taste also may be bitter.

Read relevant literature or consult a doctor for contradications, drug interactions/reactions, side-effects. Eliminate the factors that have caused this malady. Avoid recurrence by taking corrective and pre-emptive measures. Take only khichri and curd, boil drinking water. Take plenty of oral liquids coconut water, or electral powder (mixed with water and, above all, maintain and ensure highest standard of personal hygiene. Avoid eating or drinking anything outside your home.

Allopathic Treatment of Nausea/Vomiting

Branded tablets like 'Avomine'/'Domstal'/ Draminine/Ern idoxin/Gravol/Perinorm/Reglan/SiquiI/stemitel/ Tomid/ Vertin any one of the drugs can be given according to symptoms, in tablet or injection form. Normally 1-2 tablets, will suffice—given at an interval of 4-12 hours but, if an infection is given, there is hardly any need of repetition. Some drowsiness and/or sedation may also set in, hence do not drive any vehicle or operate any machinary, move out alone. The referred dose is for adults only. In case of infants, children, young and aged persons, lactating and pregnant ladies, consult your doctor for dosage and frequency, alongwith other instructions and guidelines.

If electral powder is not available, boil some water and put in a tablespoon of sugar and 1/8-1/4 tablespoon of table salt in a tumblerful of water, and let the patient drink/sip the same as frequently as needed.

Allopathic Treatment For Colic and Flatulence

- First of all take two tablets of Digene/Diovol and suck or crush them in mouth, taking some water to push the medicine down the gullet. Repeat after 2-3 hours.
- If no relief follows and pain is severe, take a capsule of Spasmo Proxyvon, 6-8 hourly. Do not use in colic of infants, children, pregnant, lactating ladies, elderly. and those having hepatic problems or Sudhinol tablet 3-4 times. (Caution is as indicated above) or Tab Tidigesic\Torolac\Walgesic\wygesic-one tablet 6 hourly.

Note: Above-mentioned medicines can also be tried in renal colic—dosage, frequency and cautions remaining the same. For further information read relevant literatures or consult your doctor. If pain and flatulence are caused by constipation, take a mild laxative or suitable drugs as suggested under 'consitpation' earlier. In any case do not ever exceed the stated dose nor/get panicky, rather wait patiently for some time, enabling the ingested medicine to act. In severe and acute case, take an injection (3 ml) of voveron which is now freely used for all types of pains, including arthritis, menstrual pains etc.

For small children and infants use only paedriatic, preparations only and never any adult dose.

Allopathic Treatment of Acidity and Heartburn

- ☞ Alkaline products can offset acidity and a tablespoon of Alkasol liquid or Alkacitron or any other such medicines will remove acidity and heartburn. Once it was told by a habitual drunkard that he mixes one or two tablespoon of alkasol with whisky and he never suffered from the two complaints. I think this may be an individual's personal experiment/opinion which might not carry medical man's nod. All the same, it may be tried when alcohol is the root cause of acidity and heartburn.
- ☞ Take two tablespoon of Digene/Polychlor forte gel/ Gelusil/Diovol straight away as soon as symptoms of acidity or heartburn appear.
- ☞ If you want to get rid of reflux oesophagitis, benign gastric duodenal ulcres/hyperacidity disorders/chronic episodic dyspepsia, Zollinger-Ellison Syndrome, take a tablet of Ranitidine (brand names Aciloc, Histac, etc.) 150 mg twice daily or 300 mg at bedtime daily for 4-8 weeks. Maintenance dose is 150 mg at bedtime. Do not stop treatment suddenly or in-between. Do not give in pregnancy, lactation, gastric malignancy, children below 12 years and infants.
- ☞ Another drug of choice is Famotidine (Brands names. Farntac, Fudone, Famonit, Farnocid, Blocacid etc.) 20/40 mg tablets. Usual dose is 20 mg at night for 4-8 weeks.

Those who are alcoholics should consult their doctor(s) about the method, dosage, safeguards, tapering of dose and or maintenance dose. Without proper guidance and know how not only the said but other medicines must never be taken.

Before concluding, the patients should try to single out the causes and try to eliminate the same. Repeated episodes of heartburn and acidity cannot be ruled out unless preventive and corrective measures are taken. Medicines can only help a patient when the patient himself is conscious about taking preventive or corrective steps but, in any case, do not expect any magical/ instant results, as it is a time-consuming complaint.

Allopathic Treatment of Peptic Ulcer

- Non absorbable antacids are preferred due to their delayed absorption. Aluminium Hydroxide (brand name: Aludrox) is the drug of choice for treatment of peptic ulcers which might cause constiption. But constipation can be removed by combining Magnesium with Aluminium. Usual dose is 200-600 mg every hour when there is acute stage but dosage and frequency may be reduced as the symptoms show a downward trend. As complete cure takes much longer time, the medicines should be continued for a month or more even when symptoms have subsided. In addition Calcium Carbonate, various Magnesium salts are available in 'Digene Gel' 'Acigon', 'Gelusil'.
- Ranitidine/Zinetac/Zanitidine/Raniten block histamine H2 receptors. Dosage is 150 mg twice daily or a single dose of 300 mg at bedtime. In order to prevent recurrence of gastric/duedenal ulcers a 150 mg dose at bed time would suffice, but has to be continued for some time.
- Another drug is 'Cimetidine' (800-1200 mg) to heal ulcer and 400 mg at bed time to prevent the recurrence of peptic ulcers but it has been ably replaced by Ranitidine which has less side effects.
- Famotidine (brand names : Famtac, Famdtin, Acipin, Fudone, Zactane) is 20 times stronger than Cimetidine and many

times stronger than Ranitidine. Its usual dose is 40 mg at bed time and has hardly much side effects.

As for side-effects, drug reactions and drug interactions, read the relevant literature or consult your doctor. These drugs must not be given up suddenly (unless there is some serious adverse effect), rather their dose should be tapered in a phased manner. Once relieved, doesn't and shouldn't mean a total immunity as there could be recurrence at any time. Cimetidine must be used with utmost care as it may decrease W.B.C.s., cause sexual dysfunction in mates, swelling in the breasts (gynaecomastia) of females. Do not take any other drug while taking Cimetidine. Rest of the drugs, not mentioned, should also not be taken without proper medical advice.

Unless dietary regimen is scruplously followed and all precipitatory factors/items omitted form diet altogether, no medicine can show any favourable and salutary results. Self-restraint and self-management, self-descipline, self-control are the well known traits for speeding up quicker recovery.

Omeprazole is reported to provide 100 percent relief after use of four weeks but in the absence of much clinical evidence, this success rate cannot be fully relied upon but other drugs, of course with requisite safeguards and cautions, may be tried with lesser side-effects.

Allopathic Treatment of Jaundice

It is mostly supportive and corrective, and medicines are generally not called for. Take tablets of liv-52 or syrup of Liv-52 (2-4 tablets thrice daily or 1-2 tablespoon thrice daily), alongwith heavy doses of Vitamin B-complex (Cap Cobadex or Cap Becosules 2-4 Capsules, daily) all after meals. Consume plenty of boiled water, coconut water, radish, papaya, sugar cane juice, curd (of toned milk) or/and whey. Avoid all types of meats, fish, spices and condiments, fats and oils (even if of unsaturated variety), tea, coffee, alcohol, tobacco, drugs and narcotics, cocoa. Juices extracted from fresh lemon and Mousambi (sweet quality only) can also be had.

Though medicines play only supportive and corrective role here. If the complaints do not yield to any method, hospitalise the patient and let him have an indoor treatment.

Diet restriction is of paramount importance. Jaundice is fully curable provided the above-mentioned points are closely followed.

Allopathic Treatment of Cirrohoris of Liver

The disease must always be treated by a qualified doctor, either at some hospital or at home, but always by a doctor and never a layman. Do not attempt any home remedies, as they simply further complicate the problem.

Auxiliary Measures

Eliminate alcohol, liquors, quinine, indigestible foods, spices, condiments and fats, milk products (except curd/whey of toned milk). Try to keep functionably of all the eliminating/excretory organs. Maintain high standard of personal hygiene and the patient be advised to take rest-in-bed but must not lead a totally sedentary life—let him have a stroll, in the morning and evening, attend to personal needs (if he can), visit the closet/bathroom.

Allopathic Treatament of Hepatitis B

It will depend upon the kind of infection imbibed and presence of symptoms. In some cases, infection is so serious as to cause death even though only 5-20 percent patients die due to such an infection.

Young infants, pregnant ladies, drug addicts, persons of weak constitution are more likely to be infected easily, though no person, or sex is immune to it. Hence, precaution is the only way to stay free of such blood transmitted infections.

Allopathic Treatment of Worms

Anti-infestive drugs are used for killing different types of worms, such as

- Pyrentel
- Piperazine
- Bepheniurn
- Diethylcarbimazine
- Niclosamide

'Pyrantel': has a neuromuscular blocking action that produces spastic paralysis in the worms. It is safe, effective and alternative to 'Mebendazole' but must be used with utmost caution as there can be liver impairment.

Piperazine': causes a flaccid paralysis of threadworms and roundworms and causes their expulsion by way of peristalsis. Both the drugs are mutually antagonistic.

'Bephenium': is an alternate drug for the treatment of round and hookworms but is poorly absorbed, hence its toxic effects are qutie rare. It is also less effective than 'Mebendazole.'

'Diethylcarbamazine': is used for treating Fialariasis but must not be used unless advised by a doctor, due to its severe hypersensitivity reactions.

Niclosamide: is an effective drug against tapeworms. It should also not be used unless a doctor advises; as it may cause vomiting/constipation.

Drug Therapy

Albendazole 400 mg tables (Trade names ABZ, Albezole, Alminth, Emanthal, Idibend, Mebex, Tagazole, Wormin, Zentel, Zumin)

Used for: Roundworm, hookworm, whipworm, tapeworm, threadworm infestations.

For Threadworms: For adults and children over 2 years400 mg (single dose only), to be followed by 100 mg dose after 2-3 weeks.

For Tapeworms: 400 mg once daily for 3 consecutive days.

For Hydatid: 400 mg. twice daily with meals for 28 days. This therapy, may be repeated after a lapse of two weeks for a total of 3 cycles.

This drug is also available in suspension form of which 5ml. suspension contains 200 mg. Dosage is the same as mentioned earlier in the case of tablets.

Note : This therapy is also an adjunct to hydated cysts or primary treatment, especially when surgery is not possible.

- Do not use in pregnancy, hormonal contraceptive, child bearing women, malfunctioning of liver, breast-feeding.
- It may cause headache, gastro-intestinal disturbances, fever, rashes, dizziness, alopecia (baldness), convulsions and meningism in cerebral disease.

Now-a-days only a single drug treatment is given for all the worm infections and it is quite convenient also for the patient.

Auxiliary Measures

- Clip nails of hands and feet and keep them clean.
- Before going, coming back, before and after eating, after defecation wash hands with soap.
- Wash thoroughly all fruits and vegetables.
- Take plenty of roughage to ward off chances of any constipation.
- Observe yourself and also educate children about personal hygiene.
- Ensure that the cooks and servants also observe requisite level of cleanliness and personal hygiene.
- Do not eat/drink any foodstuff which is exposed to dust, flies, insects, is impure and contaminated, stale, foul smelling or rotten.

Allopathic Treatment of Cancer of Stomach

Operation is the only option left, but chances of full recovery are not very encouraging. Anyway, one has to take a chance of operation, when no other option is left.

Allopathic Treatment of Piles

Liquid Cremaffin. 1 tablespoon should be taken at night before retiring to bed, otherwise mix 1-2 tablespoon of Isapgol husk to milk which should be taken at bedtime. Locally apply ointment anovate or proctodsedyl in the rectum with the applicator at night, before and after defecation (each time) so as to facilitate smooth passage of stools or use rectal capsules of proctosedyl-M. Main emphasis should be to ensure smooth passage of stools. In some persons hypersensitivity to the ingredients may cause some problems in which condition stop using the local ointment etc., and consult your doctor.

■

15

PHYSICAL ACTIVITIES—TO CURE DIFFERENT DIGESTIVE DISORDERS

Physical activities provide good circulation, physical strength and stamina and a supple body.

Cardiovascular endurance is the ability of the heart, blood vessels and blood to carry oxygen to the cells and to carry waste products away from them. Muscular endurance is the capability of muscles to maintain repeated exercise and muscular strength is a capacity to carry, lift, push or pull a heavy load. Flexibility is the ability of joints to move through their full range of motion-they will not move easily.

Optimum Heart-Rate

Your optimum heart-rate during exercise should ideally be kept at 60-80 percent of your maximum heart-rate, which you can establish by subtracting your age. People who exercise regularly learn what their optimum heart-rate feels like. As you become fitter, you will need to step up the intensity of exercise to maintain your optimum heart- rate.

To calculate heart-rate, place two fingers on the pulse at the side of your neck or on your wrist. Count the beats for 15 seconds, and then multiply the number by four.

Cycling: gives the heart and blood circulation a thorough work-out without straining the joints. It is an excellent way of getting fresh air, but a stationary bicycle indoors might be more practical for some people.

Dancing: exercises the heart, lungs and muscles, and the social aspect is an added bonus. Choose from tango, salsa, jazz, ballet or any other form of energetic dance.

Downhill skiing: Helps develop balance, agility and coordination, while cross-country skiing provides a more complete aerobic workout and exercise, more muscle groups than any other sport.

Fit for life: Physical fitness requires cardiovascular endurance, muscular endurance and strength, and flexibility. Taking 20-30 minutes aerobic exercise (3-5 times a week) brings definite health benefits.

Cardiovascular: Endurance is developed by vigorous aerobic exercise, such as jogging, sustained for at least 12 minutes without a break (you should be puffing but not so hard that you can't carry on a conversation). Aerobic exercise oxygenates the muscles and enables the heart to pump more efficiently.

Muscular: Endurance is built up with repeated exercising of large muscle groups, as in swimming.

Muscular strength is developed with anaerobic exercise, as in weight lifting or tennis, which consists of brief busts of intense activity.

Flexibility is achieved by stretching muscles and is maintained by activities such as golf or yoga. It stops connective tissue shortening and tightening, prevents muscles being pulled or torn, relieves pain, boosts muscle strength and tone, and helps prevent injury. Flexibility can enhance body awareness and appearance, increase energy and improves circulation.

Which Activity?

It is a fact that if you enjoy a form of exercise, you are more likely to stick with it. It prevents boredom by varying exercises for example, try skipping sometimes instead of running.

Walking, which has a host of health benefits, can easily be incorporated into a daily routine.

Tennis is good for agility and co-ordination, and helps build up muscular strength.

Running or jogging is the aerobic exercise par excellence, but don't attempt it until you can walk briskly for 3 km (2 miles) without difficulty. Always wear well-cushioned shoes that bend at the ball of the foot.

Exercise classes vary from stretching and weight training to step aerobics, jazz, dance and dynamic yoga.

In his famous book entitled 'Natural Living' Mark Eve has mentioned following sports related activities.

1. Badminton
2. Golf
3. Jogging (Aerobic) or Running
4. Tennis (Aerobic)
5. Brisk walking (Aerobic)
6. Cycling (Aerobic)
7. Skipping (Aerobic)
8. Swimming (Aerobic)
9. Football (Aerobic)
10. Boxing
11. Volley Ball
12. Squash
13. Rebounding (Aerobic)
14. Dancing
15. Jazz dance
16. Gardening

There could be and are other types of activities to maintain general good health, for instanced Kabaddi, Kho-Kho, Wrestling etc. In their book entitled ' Encyclopaedia of Complementary Mundane' Anne Woodham and Dr. David Peters have suggested some excellent tips on general upkeep of sound health.

I have stated earlier that dwarfism is the cause of multiple factors which, when combined together, prove as retarding and inhibitory factors, out of which balanced diet, proper activity and rest are the three major ingredients and entire health will be thrown out of gear if one aspect is scarified or over-emphasized for the other one or when proper balance is not maintained.

Deviating from the main topic I will suggest that all persons, whether young or old, should ask themselves following questions and decide for yourself where you actually stand when following health problem related questions are asked:

1. Are you physically fit enough to do the things you want to?
2. Do you get all the sleep you need?
3. Do you exercise for at least 20-30 minutes, three times a day?
4. Do you give yourself enough time to warm up and cool down before and after exercising?
5. Are you comfortable with your weight, shape and physical condition?
6. Given the option, do you walk or use the stairs?
8. Are you well enough to work everyday?
9. Do you feel secure and satisfied in what you do?
10. Is your environment free from pollution (of air, noise, chemically)?
11. Do you feel in control of your workload?
12. Do you take enough breaks during the day to keep your mind alert and reduce body tension?
13. Do you drink more than three times a day or do you use rotationally dangerous recreational things?

14. Do you suffer from high blood pressure, raised blood cholesterol, diabetes; had an attack (of heart) before 40, gout, blood cancer, glaucoma, and bowl cancer?
15. Do you have a periodical check up which includes x-rays, blood tests, urine and stool tests, eye-nose, ear and throat tests?
16. Do you take care of abnormal and/or unusual growths on/in your body?
17. Do you find it difficult to enjoy/relaxes moments of pleasure or you simply and easily buckle under stressful conditions?
18. Do you become panicky in an unfavourable situation or blame others for your faults also?
19. Do you take a wholesome diet daily and affect occasional changes in your menu?
20. Do you avoid junk and processed food?
21. Do you drink enough fluids to keep your urine light pale?
22. Do you often skip meals or every time is a mealtime for you.
23. Does any change in dress, diet, environs, house, job or friends impact your life?
24. Do you take out some moments to relax?
25. Do you get 6-8 hours sleep daily?

If your response to the above questions is in the negative, you need to assess your life, living pattern, habits eating habits, with suitable and requisite changes failing which life may seem to be a burden for you. Self-assessment and drawing a self balance sheet are not easy tasks but when there is an honest approach and strong will and determination, most of the said problems could be easily surmounted and tied over.

Sports and Games—as a means to Shed Weight

Badminton

If played in singles it exhausts whole body. It induces sweating, sheds extra weight, strengthens bones, bone joints, muscles, suppleness and imparts glow to skin. You need an equally able partner to fit in the slot.

Tennis

It is more vigorous game than Badminton and players attain bony and muscular strength by felling trees with an axe. If you can play tennis daily for 30-60 minutes, you can achieve far more than you can aspire to achieve from badminton. Persons with weak bones and muscles are considered unfit for this game. Here also singles game is more beneficial.

Golf

It is game of the elite class and is played more as a social status than for much for health gain. Here the movement is quite slow. The only advantage, if at all, is to walk down to pick up the ball. Even muscle development is slow.

Running or Jogging

Do not straight away jump on to jogging. To begin with cultivate habit of walking briskly for 3 kms, without any problem. Distance should be added daily so as to gradually reach the 3 km. mark. Wear well-cushioned shoes that bend at (point of) ball of the foot. Running will enable you to build up resistance in a graduated manner. Control over respiration, not getting tired or develop pain or ache are the prerequisites to jogging. Persons who suffer from some cardiac problem, high blood pressure, weak joints, asthma should take to jogging only after getting clearance from concerned expert. Jogging or brisk running exercise whole of the body and can help in adding to height but it requires highly nutritious diet. If food does not match the quantum of jogging activity, it may prove even harmful and counter- productive. Jogging should be on toes and not on heels but if it is otherwise, it is simply walking and not jogging.

Cycling

Cycling is meant to enhance cardiac output, tone up and strengthen bones, muscles of legs, but doesn't exercise any ankles and feet. Cycling is a good exercise if done on the open roads so as to inhale fresh air. But in some cases indoor cycling gives the heart and circulation a thorough workout without straining the involved joints. Cycling is an ideal substitute for those who cannot jog or run or even walk briskly, running jogging and cycling must not be practised soon after taking meals. If you want to reach the paddles, but refrain from bending your body to one side while trying to reach the paddle. Height of seat can be adjusted as per need of an individual. If you have any problem in gripping, you should use a static cycle, preferably with an adjustable weight attached therewith- it will help to strengthen thighs, knees and femur.

Unless there is some physical disability cycling is an excellent exercise for all age groups of both sexes. Accelerate speed and once you have picked up the desired speed, you should try to maintain the built up momentum. If you wish, you can have a speedometer affixed to your cycle so as to know at what speed you are moving the wheels.

Skipping

This is an excellent aerobic exercise to enhance height and reduce weight. Use a strong but flexible rope for the purpose and with the help of your hands, move the same in a circular form from head to feet. You should skip when the rope passes from beneath your feet. Skip on toes and do not let heels touch the grounds. Momentum, once built up, should be maintained uniformly. If you get tired start panting, do not push skipping exercise any further. Tiredness during exercise is the nature's warning signal, demanding you to stop the exercise forthwith.

Some persons keep on running while skipping but it requires practice.

If skipping with a rope poses any problem, you can skip at the same place, by keeping your hands on the waist. Skipping exercises and activates entire body and if you practice it, you do not have to take to any other exercise. Start by skipping for 2 minutes with 10- minute break and also increase the repetitions gradually raising to 30 seconds. Thus doing 3 skipping sets for 30 seconds with a 5-minutes break.

Swimming

It is an excellent aerobic exercise but one has to learn the art of swimming from a coach. Swimming exercises whole body, expands chest, improves respiration, pushes up circulation, strengthens bones and muscles, and imparts suppleness. Never venture into swimming without accompaniment of a coach otherwise it may prove fatal. Swimming is one of the best and fastest of aerobics to boost overall fitness, muscles tone, joint flexibility and relaxation. Use head- gear, earplugs, and goggles so as to prevent entry of water. Do 4 lengths of a 25 meter pool, rest for a minute and try to build endurance by reducing rest time and increasing time of swimming and within 15 days you will find yourself in a better frame. An hour's breast- stroke burns 500-800 calories.

Football

It is good exercise for the legs that may get lengthened, muscles stretched, connective tissue shortening and tightening stopped. It also prevents from muscle being torn or pulled, relieves pain, boosts up strength of (leg) muscles but injuries may be sustained during playing the game.

Hockey

It has some added advantage over football because upper parts of body are also equally benefited by brisk stick play. Chances of injuries are far greater and if caution is thrown to winds one may sustain even serious injuries, especially to feet, ankles, toes knees and hands. Slow movements is not possible in both football and hockey sports. But, more players get injured during hockey playing than football. It is a far brisk and fast sport than football; hence the players should be extra careful in avoiding chances of serious and damaging injuries.

Cricket

It doesn't exercise whole body and is a slow game as compared to football, hockey, tennis and badminton, though chances of injury are quite frequent and any part of body may get injured. Head injury, chest and rib-cage injury, injury to hands, forearm and knees are quite common and some of which may cause fatality even. Only the fieldsmen, who have to run quite fast, get aerobic benefit. The fast bowlers have added advantage over slow bowlers. Cricket is not a sport where all the players can be equally benefited, as whole body doesn't get involved. If you are waiting for your chance.

Dancing

Ballroom dances are leisure dances and have no significant role in exercise. Swinging, hip-swinging dances, dance of Indian style, twist, shake are good exercise which can prove useful but these disciplines have been turned into professionalism, hence majority of people cannot benefit. If you can twist even for 3-5 minutes whole body will derive benefit but it carries some risks also and that may be the reason why the same is becoming rare these days. Indian dances are more scientific. They tone up entire body, strengthen muscles and build up general resistance of the body. Bhangra of Punjab is an all round excellent dance where all body parts get exercised, toned up and rejuvenated. Some of the regional dances are far easier to perform, cost effective and rewarding and infuse new life into entire body without much wastage of time, money and energy.

Walking

It has host of health benefits and does not require any extra effort except, of course, your will determination and persistence. If you are walking with a partner, walking can be more rewarding, enjoyable and communicative. Brisk walking is required in the morning, preferably before sunrise. You should wear sports/walking shoes that do not tire or pain your feet. Evening walk should simply be a stroll. You can add speed to walking but it should in a gradual way. Walking may/may not add to your height but will have salutary effect on general well being, digestion, respiration and suppleness. Do not smoke, eat or drink before, during or immediately after walking. A glass of hot milk, say after 15-30 minutes of walking, will give you added and extra energy. You cannot burn much of calories by slow walking but you can do so by brisk walking.

Aerobic excercises

- Start with 10 minutes of light to moderat exercise. Work it up- at-least 30 minutes a day with a month. For even greater benefits, and perhaps to prolong your life, build up to a regimen of more vigorous exercise. If you get strapped for time, remember, your 30 minutes don,t have to be consecutive.
- When you start, do so slowly. Limber up by doing light excercise that straight your muscles slowly and gently. Similarly, after you have completed your main workout, allow yourself a "cool down" period. Wait a while and get back your noarmal rate of pulse before you drink water or jump into a hot shower.
- Restrict outdoor schedules to early morning or evening when the smog and pollution levels are at their lowest. Running on polluted road, inhaling the carbon monoxide, will be counter-productive.
- Find an excercise you will enjoy, not simply endure. Tune in to the sensual aspects of the excercise.

- Do regular deep-breathing excercise five minutes before and after your workout. This provides the body with extra oxygen. It also increases lung capacity. A few minutes at an open window each day or measured breathing while walking will suffice to relax the body and the mind.
- Follow this 5-minutes period of deep breathing with another 5-minute period of relaxation. The yogic shavasana—lying flat on your back on the flor-performed after exercise helps relax and smoothe the body, besides dispelling negative emotions, depression and lethargy.
- Set Realistic goals. Don't get derailed by excuses. Keep in mind that the days you feel least eneretic and eager to exercise are exactly when you need it the most. Far from including fatigue, a regular workout, once made a habit, will not only improve stamina but will also invigorate you, sending a rush of blood into the forearms and the legs.
- Don't push too hard. Never overstrain your muscles. If you feel you cannot exert yourself any longer, espically while doing aerobics, or if you feel breathless and dizzy or feel a tightness or pain in the chest, stop exercising immediately and consult your physician for some less strenuous mode of working out. All you really need to do is push hard enough to work up a fine sheen of sweat and raise your heart rate above its usual level.

■

16

CALORIES, HEIGHT-WEIGHT AND ESSENTIAL NUTRIENTS TABLES

Table of Calories Burn in Physical Activities

In the following table an effort has been made to spell out calories spent by an individual in relation to his/her physical activity (For all sexes and age-groups).

	Activity	Calories expended per hours
(i)	**Light Activity**	**50-200 Calories's Group**
	Lying down/ sleeping	80
	Sitting	100
	Driving a Car	120
	Household work	180
(ii)	**Moderate Activity**	**200-300 Calories's Group**
	Bicycling (8.25 kms)	210
	Walking (4.25 kms)	210
	Gardening	220
	Canoeing (4.25 kms)	230
	Golf	250
	Lawn-Mowing (Power mover)	250
	Lawn-Mowing (Hand Mover)	270
	Bowling	270

(iii)	**Marked Activity**	**300-400 Calories's Group**
	Walking (6 kms)	300
	Swimming (40 Mtrs.)	300
	Rowing (4.25 kms)	300
	Fencing	300
	Badminton	350
	Horse-Riding (Trotting)	350
	Roller-Skating	350
	Volley Ball	350
	Square Dancing	350
	Table-Tannis	360
(iv)	**Vigorous Activity**	**Over 400 Calories's Group**
	Ice-skating (16 kms)	400
	Sawing or wood-chopping	400
	Tennis	420
	Hill-climbing	480
	Skying	490
	Hand ball	600
	Bicycling (21 kms)	600
	Running (16 kms)	900

Table of Daily Calorie Requirements (during 24 hours)

Age Group	*Calorie Requirements*
upto 6 months	120 Calories per kg body weight
7-12 months	100 Calories per kg body weight
1-3 years	1200 Calories
4-6 years	1500 Calories

7-9 years	1800 Calories
10-12 years	2100 Calories
13-15 years (boys)	2500 Calories
13-15 years (girls)	2200 Calories
16-18 years (boys)	3000 Calories
16-18 years (girls)	2200 Calories
Men, doing light work	2200 Calories
Men, doing medium work	2800 Calories
Men, doing heavy work	3400 Calories
Women, doing light work	1900 Calories
Women, doing medium work	2200 Calories
Women, doing heavy work	2800 Calories

Note—Parameters shown above are merely indicative of general standards but calories for each person are required to be worked out on the basis of age, sex, amount of manual labour put in, health status, person's height, weight and climate of a place.

Daily Calorie According to Body Weight and Activity

(Daily Calorie Requirement in Food)
(Per kg Body Weight)

Weight of a Person	Office Workers (Light Work)	Medium Work	Hard Work
Under weight	35	40	45
Normal weight	30	35	40
Overweight	20	25	30

Note—For athletes, sports persons, persons engaged in strenuous work, growing children, pregnant women and men with malnutrition, calorie requirement should be measured in relation to physical condition and the amount of calories expended or expected to be spent. Each case has, naturally, to be individualised because no two cases could be identical. Since weight also must commensurate with height of a person and, in keeping with requirements of these two factors, following table will give an idea as to whether a person's weight is in proportion to his height.

Table of Ideal Body Weight in Kgs. and Height in Cms

Height (in cms)	Age Groups 18-20	23-27	28-32	33-37
	(Weight in kgs)			
150	45.5	47.0	48.3	49.4
152	46.2	47.8	49.7	50.4
154	47.1	48.7	50.3	51.4
156	48.0	49.7	51.4	52.6
158	49.5	50.8	52.5	53.7
160	50.0	52.0	53.7	54.9
162	51.2	53.2	54.9	56.1
164	52.4	54.4	56.2	57.2
166	53.7	55.7	57.6	59.0
168	55.1	57.2	59.9	60.0
170	56.5	58.7	60.6	62.2
172	58.2	60.2	62.1	63.9
174	59.5	61.7	63.7	65.6
176	61.0	63.3	65.3	67.3
178	62.5	64.9	67.0	69.00
180	64.1	66.5	68.7	70.7
182	65.7	68.1	70.4	72.4
184	67.3	69.7	72.1	74.1
186	68.9	71.4	73.8	75.8
188	70.5	73.1	75.6	77.8
190	72.1	74.8	77.4	79.6

Height (in cms)	Age Groups 38-42	43-47	48-52	Above 53 years
150	49.8	50.1	50.3	50.5
152	50.8	51.1	51.3	51.5
154	51.9	52.2	52.4	52.1
156	53.0	53.3	53.6	53.7
158	54.1	54.4	54.7	54.9
160	55.3	55.7	56.0	56.3
162	56.6	57.0	57.4	57.7
164	58.0	58.5	58.9	59.2
166	59.5	60.0	60.4	60.8
168	61.1	61.6	62.0	62.4
170	62.8	63.2	63.7	64.1
172	64.5	65.0	65.5	65.9
174	66.2	66.7	67.3	67.7
176	67.9	68.4	69.1	69.5
178	69.6	70.2	70.9	71.3
180	71.3	72.0	72.9	73.2
182	73.0	73.8	74.5	75.1
184	74.8	75.6	76.3	77.0
186	76.6	77.4	78.1	78.9
188	78.4	79.2	79.9	80.8
190	80.2	81.0	81.7	82.7

Note: ± 5 percent weight should be taken as normal weight or, to be precise, marginally high/average weight. But ± 15-20 percent weight, over and above the ideal weight, should be considered as 'overweight' and the latter calls for a guarded and modified approach in tapering and slashing down calories but, care should be taken that calories are not reduced to such an extent that a person gets weaker and is not in a fit frame to discharge even his normal chores.

Table of Daily Average Requirement of Essential Nutrients

Vitamins		*Daily Requirement*
'A'	(For Normal Person)	5000 I.U.
	(For Pregnant Women)	8000 I.U.
B-1 (Thiamine)		1.25 mg
B-2 (Riboflavin)		1.50 mg
B-6 (Pyridoxine)		2.00 mg
B-12 (Cobalamin)		6.00 mg
Niacin (Nictoinamide)		20 mg
B-5 (Pentatonic Acid)		10 mg
Botanic and Folic acid		0.31 mg
Vitamin-C (Ascorbic Acid)		60 mg
Vitamin-D (Calciferol)		400 - I.U.
Vitamin-E (Tocopherol)		30 I.U.-400 I.U.
Vitamin-F		Not clear
Vitamin-K (depending on clotting condition)		S.O.S.
Vitamin-P (Bioflavonoid)		Not clear
Minerals and Trace Elements		
Calcium	For growing children	500-800 mg
Calcium	For nursing /lactating mothers	1000-1400 mg
Calcium	For Adults	400-500 mg
Chromium		1-2 mg
Copper		2 mg
Iron		12-15 mg

Iodine	.01 - .02 mg
Manganese	5 mg
Magnesium	200-400 mg
Phosphorus	1 mg
Potassium	1000-4000 mgm (1-4 gms)
Sodium	400-1500 mgm
Selenium	50-200 mgm
Zinc	10-15 mg

Note—The aforesaid details are based on daily requirements of a normal and healthy person and are, thus, general and not particular indications. Every case has different expenditure, health status/diseased conditions, age, sex, regional climate, availability of recommended food items, and capacity of a person to purchase. In short, all efforts should be made to derive energy from available natural sources, such as vegetables, sea-foods (including fish), grain cereals, natural water resources, animal foods and products (like milk, butter, clarified butter, cheese, whey etc.), poultry products. As far as possible, try to avoid branded and commercial products and medicines, tinned and exposed foods etc. Emphasis ought to be on quality of the food but never on the quantity.

■■■